TASTE

THE INFOGRAPHIC BOOK OF FOOD

LAURA ROWE

TASTE

THE INFOGRAPHIC BOOK OF FOOD

LAURA ROWE

Aurum
Press

First published in Great Britain
2015 by Aurum Press Ltd
74-77 White Lion Street
London N1 9PF
www.aurumpress.co.uk

A catalogue record for this book is available
from the British Library.

ISBN 978 1 78131 463 0

1 3 5 7 9 10 8 6 4 2
2015 2017 2019 2018 2016

Typeset in Tabac Slab by Vicki Turner.
Printed in China

With thanks to...

—

Although I write every single day for a living, there's something incredibly special about having penned a book. In an age where everything is in the cloud, and is as quickly forgotten from our feeds as it was originally written, having a real-life, tangible book, that can still be picked up, touched, smelled, used as a coffee cup coaster, dust gatherer and thing that people can read is, actually, amazing. It's an opportunity for which I will be forever grateful.

So firstly, I'd like to thank Melissa, for a great idea, for believing in me, and her support and praise. I'd also like to apologise – I'm sorry for the stress! To Vicki, for bringing my words to life with her beautiful illustrations and her constant cheery disposition. Karen and Rob, thanks for dragging us to the finish line. Jon, Jess and Ben: much obliged for your expertise.

Then there are those that have put up with me for the past year. Kate – flatmate, work wife and best friend – thank you for looking after me, cooking me dinner, and all the meats. To my besties, whose constant motivation, support, and food-and-drink care packages have kept me going: Meg, Rosie, Sam, Mary – you are the best. To mates I have neglected, forgive me.

To mum and dad, I hope I've made you proud. I love you. And Lukey, thank you for being consistently uninterested. To bears and hummingbirds, you are very special to me.

TASTE: CONTENTS

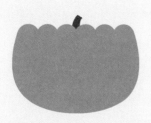

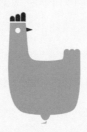

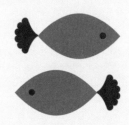

FROM THE PLOT

OFF THE FARM

OUT THE WATER

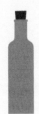

IN THE LARDER

ON THE TABLE

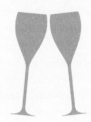

FROM THE BAR

ANY OTHER BUSINESS

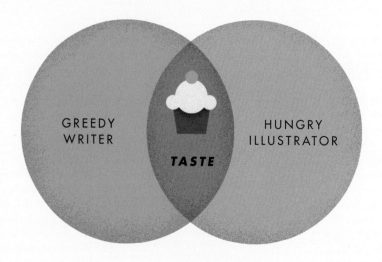

GREEDY WRITER

HUNGRY ILLUSTRATOR

TASTE

TASTE

By Laura Rowe

A few years ago I spotted an infographic that estimated we consume up to 285 pieces of content just through social media every day. And I could believe it. When I wake up, the first thing I do is check Twitter; as I walk to work I read emails; and before I've even finished brewing my first cup of tea, I will have scanned the headlines. My life is all about information consumption – and food consumption, a *lot* of food consumption.

I'm a food writer, but first and foremost I've always been hungry for knowledge (admittedly that could be on how to make the ultimate cheese toastie). So infographics – where information is condensed and presented in a visual way – have always appealed. They're a quick, easy (and often more fun) way of digesting stats, facts and subjects that would otherwise take hours to research. Information suddenly becomes bitesize.

So what exactly is an infographic? It's the question I've answered most when describing

this book to friends and family as I explain where I've been hiding for the past year. It's as simple as it sounds: information presented in a graphic way. We don't have time to digest tomes on our favourite subjects. We want to know it all, and we want to know it now, quickly and efficiently. And an infographic helps you do just that. It breaks down big subjects, making them accessible and understandable. Someone else has done all the hard work for you.

There are infographics on facial hair shapes, on the circles of hell in Dante's *Inferno*, on the dunkability of biscuits. There are even infographics on infographics. This, though, is meant to be a collection of illustrations that will help you be a better cook and diner. You see, this is an infographic book of food. An exploration of taste – from the ingredients we cook with, to the dishes we eat – around the world.

Each of the illustrations have been chosen for their international relevance, whether through popular culture (the burger), tradition

(Christmas lunch) or social importance (salt). I've broken them down into easy-to-find categories too, starting with ingredients 'From the Plot', plucked from earth or branch; to foodstuffs 'Off the Farm' or 'Out the Water'.

There are chapters on your favourite storecupboard essentials within 'In the Larder', and the meals (sweet and savoury) that you must try in 'On the Table'. I've also briefly touched on a few of the world's most important drinks in 'From the Bar', including beer, cider and wine; tea, coffee and cordials; right through to the old favourite, gin. And, there are some infographics that every foodie, whether they be a keen cook, eater or both, should know in 'Any Other Business'. Ever read a recipe and not known how many grams equate to a pound? Or what time of year you should be eating asparagus? Or what knives to stock in your culinary arsenal? This is the section for you.

There are flow diagrams and pie charts, Venn diagrams and recipes, step-by-steps and timelines, spider diagrams and actual spiders (they're considered a food by some!). There's even a sausage solar system. You can sit down and read it all in one go munching through every last morsel. Or, you can dip in and out, and share with friends, like a table overflowing with tapas and the finest sherry.

Taste is meant to be a starting point, a beginner's guide to being a foodie. Think of it as an *amuse bouche*, a tasty tidbit to whet your appetite to eat more and learn more. This is the sort of book you'll keep by your bedside for when you can't sleep (eating sheep is so much more fun than counting them, after all). It'll be the book you lay on your coffee table and test your friends' knowledge with. It's a resource and a play thing. It's the gift you can give to anyone. We do all eat, after all.

On a personal level, this has been a crash course in a subject I thought I knew pretty well already. But that's the amazing thing about food. There's always a new tip to pick up, a trick to learn, or a history to discover. It's a world of innovation, creativity and colour.

It's made me a million times better at my day job, as an editor of an award-winning food magazine in the South West of England, and hungrier than ever. I've scoured the internet, trawled my vast cookery book collection, and been back to the library more than I ever did at university. While I've tried to be as authoritative as possible, as with any of my articles or blog posts, I hope you get a flavour of my personality, too. Food doesn't have to be serious, or worthy; it is meant to be fun and enjoyable.

Happy reading; I hope you enjoy this information-packed book about beloved food as much as I enjoyed writing it.

Now if you'll excuse me, I've got dinner to make...

A SNAFFLE MAIDEN'S ESSENTIAL GUIDE TO A YEAR'S WORTH OF BOOK WRITING

You will need to consume...

1,148 biscuits

1,095 cups of tea

372 cans of Diet Coke

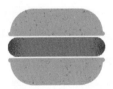

79 macarons
(12 of which were perfect, the rest we won't talk about)

41 blocks of Cheddar

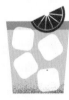

200 gin and tonics*

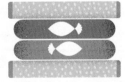

6 fish finger sandwiches

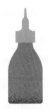

3 bottles of Sriracha

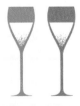

1 bottle of Champagne
(to celebrate)

*Okay, you caught me out. Make that 298

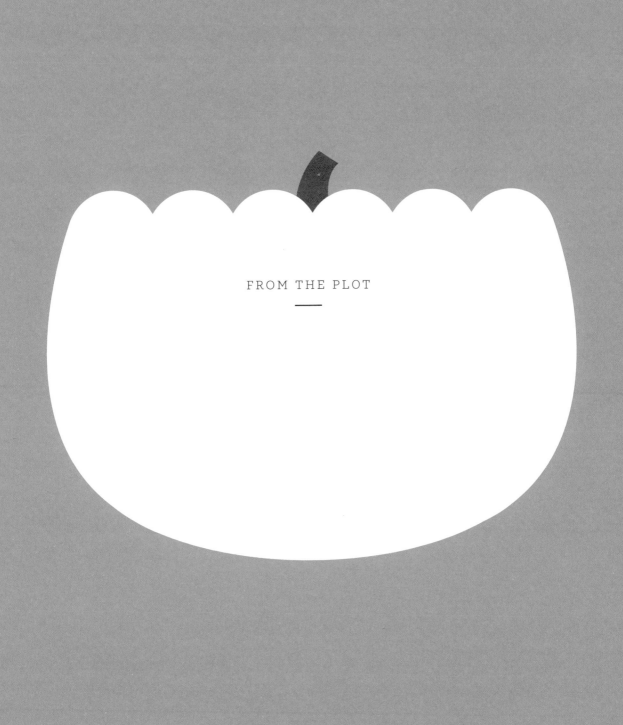

FROM THE PLOT

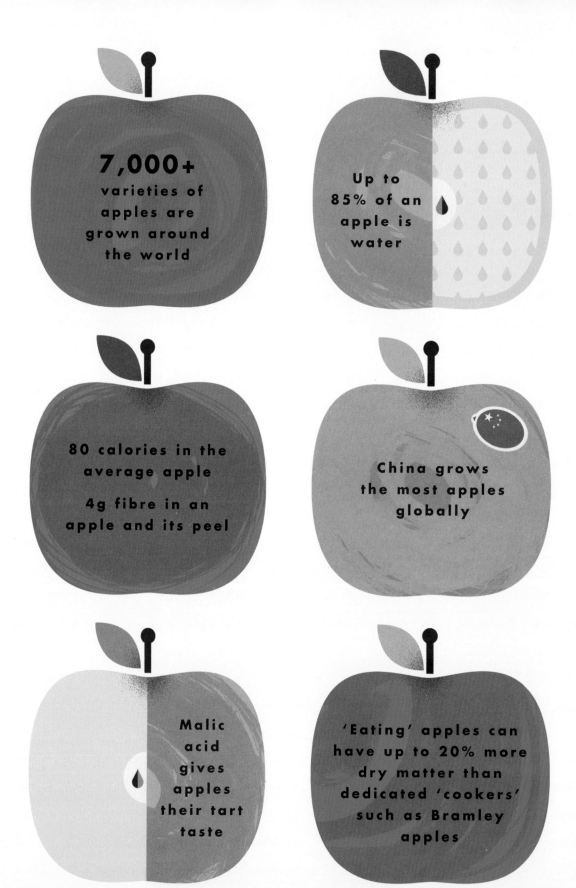

7,000+ varieties of apples are grown around the world

Up to **85%** of an apple is water

80 calories in the average apple

4g fibre in an apple and its peel

China grows the most apples globally

Malic acid gives apples their tart taste

'Eating' apples can have up to 20% more dry matter than dedicated 'cookers' such as Bramley apples

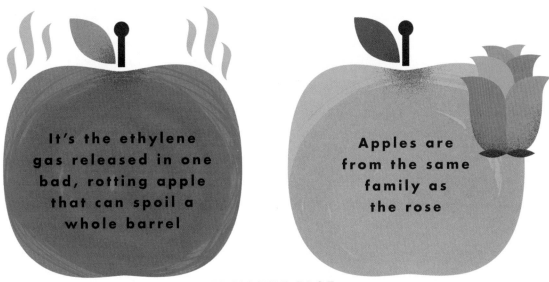

It's the ethylene gas released in one bad, rotting apple that can spoil a whole barrel

Apples are from the same family as the rose

APPLE: ALL IN THE BITE

The humble apple – that staple of our fruit bowl, with promises that one a day will keep the doctor away – has played a rather significant role throughout history. It's the forbidden fruit that tempted Eve in the Garden of Eden; it represented love, fertility and youthfulness in much Greek and Norse mythology; and Isaac Newton stumbled across the concept of gravity with the help of a falling apple.

They're best grown in temperate zones but varieties in all shades of red, yellow and green are harvested. Australia has produced some of the globe's most popular eating apples – from long-growing, sweet Pink Lady (also known as Cripps Pink) to the green, sharp and crunchy Granny Smith. Britain, meanwhile, is the only country to grow apples specifically for cooking; namely, the Bramley. With its high concentration of malic acid compared to sugar, it has a stronger, sharper apple flavour that sticks around after cooking.

Apples can be round, flat, oblong or conical in shape, and generally have creamy, white flesh – except for the modern German strain Baya Marisa (also known as Tickled Pink), that has a striking flash of red. And don't be confused by the recently developed 'papple', which started appearing in 2012 thanks to New Zealand growers. It's actually a hybrid of European and Asian pear varieties and no relation to the apple at all.

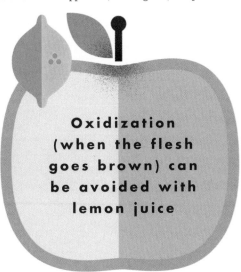

Oxidization (when the flesh goes brown) can be avoided with lemon juice

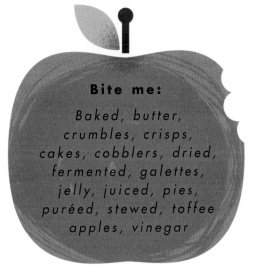

Bite me:

Baked, butter, crumbles, crisps, cakes, cobblers, dried, fermented, galettes, jelly, juiced, pies, puréed, stewed, toffee apples, vinegar

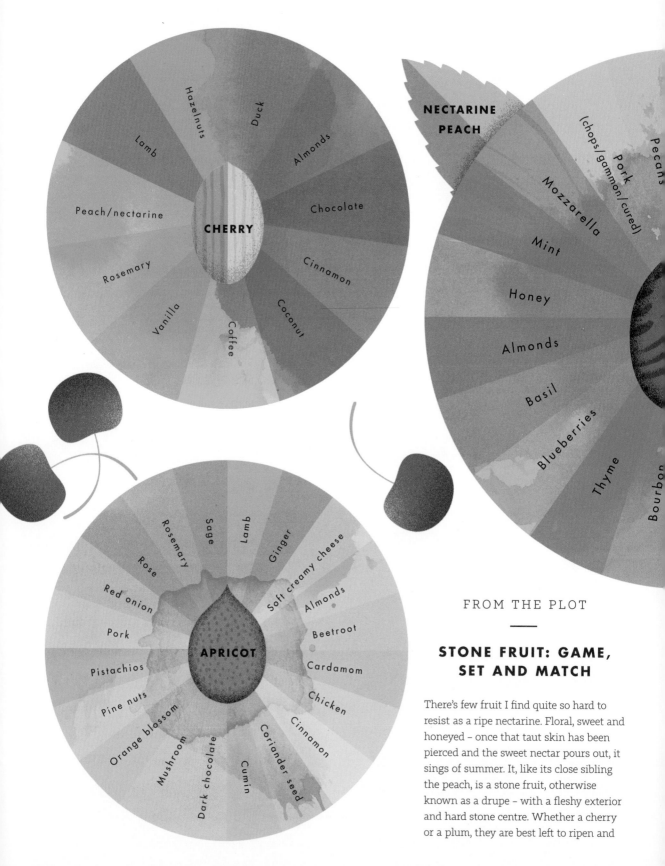

CHERRY

Hazelnuts
Duck
Almonds
Chocolate
Cinnamon
Coconut
Coffee
Vanilla
Rosemary
Peach/nectarine
Lamb

NECTARINE PEACH

Pecans
Pork (chops/gammon/cured)
Mozzarella
Mint
Honey
Almonds
Basil
Blueberries
Thyme
Bourbon

APRICOT

Sage
Lamb
Ginger
Soft creamy cheese
Almonds
Beetroot
Cardamom
Chicken
Cinnamon
Coriander seed
Cumin
Dark chocolate
Mushroom
Orange blossom
Pine nuts
Pistachios
Pork
Red onion
Rose
Rosemary

FROM THE PLOT

—

STONE FRUIT: GAME, SET AND MATCH

There's few fruit I find quite so hard to
resist as a ripe nectarine. Floral, sweet and
honeyed – once that taut skin has been
pierced and the sweet nectar pours out, it
sings of summer. It, like its close sibling
the peach, is a stone fruit, otherwise
known as a drupe – with a fleshy exterior
and hard stone centre. Whether a cherry
or a plum, they are best left to ripen and

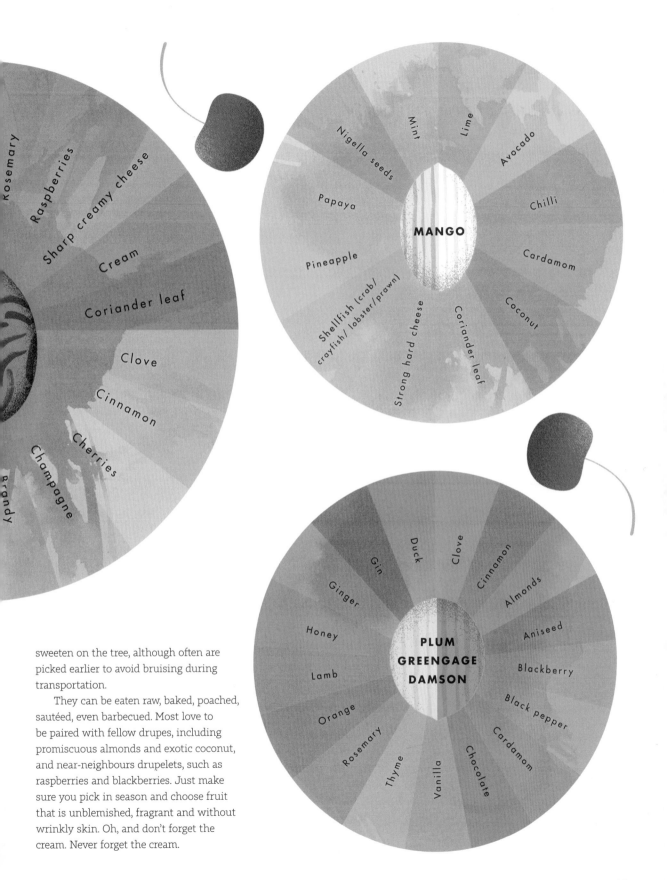

MANGO

Mint
Lime
Avocado
Chilli
Cardamom
Coconut
Coriander leaf
Strong hard cheese
Shellfish (crab/crayfish/lobster/prawn)
Pineapple
Papaya
Nigella seeds

Rosemary
Raspberries
Sharp creamy cheese
Cream
Coriander leaf
Clove
Cinnamon
Cherries
Champagne
Brandy

PLUM GREENGAGE DAMSON

Duck
Clove
Cinnamon
Almonds
Aniseed
Blackberry
Black pepper
Cardamom
Chocolate
Vanilla
Thyme
Rosemary
Orange
Lamb
Honey
Ginger
Gin

sweeten on the tree, although often are picked earlier to avoid bruising during transportation.

They can be eaten raw, baked, poached, sautéed, even barbecued. Most love to be paired with fellow drupes, including promiscuous almonds and exotic coconut, and near-neighbours drupelets, such as raspberries and blackberries. Just make sure you pick in season and choose fruit that is unblemished, fragrant and without wrinkly skin. Oh, and don't forget the cream. Never forget the cream.

SWEET

- Posset
- Curd
- Soufflé
- Pancakes
- Tarte au citron
- Meringue pie
- Cheesecake
- Frozen (granita, sorbet)
- Mousse
- Turkish delight
- Cake (drizzle, pound, muffins)
- Biscuits

SAVOURY

Chinese lemon chicken

Avgolemono
(Greek lemon, chicken, rice and egg soup)

STAR DISH

FROM THE PLOT

LEMON: FIX UP, LOOK SHARP

For something that is essentially inedible raw – causing cheeks to pucker and eyes to wince – it is remarkable how important lemon is in the kitchen. It can be used in sweet and savoury dishes alike. Its fragrant zest is as useful as its acidic juice (although be sure to avoid the bitter white pith).

PAIR WITH

- Cream cheese
- Almonds
- Egg
- Honey
- Asparagus
- Poppy seeds
- Lavender
- Fennel
- Pasta
- Artichokes
- Butter
- Olives
- Saffron
- Rice and grains
- Cream
- Lime
- Blueberries
- Potatoes
- Chicken
- Soft & woody herbs
- Chilli
- Ginger
- Garlic
- Raspberries
- Shellfish & fish
- Capers

ONE LEMON
=
Citric acid & pectin
2-3 tbsp juice
Vitamin C

16

CLEAN

- Deodorize fridge & microwave
- Wipe chopping boards
- Shine aluminium pans

SEASON

- Use juice like salt or pepper to flavour a dish
- Vinaigrette
- Gremolata (zest, garlic, parsley)
- Preserved lemons with salt
- Marinade

GET SCIENTIFIC

- Slowing oxidization (discoloration)
- Tenderize meat
- 'Cook' fish in a ceviche

A simple slice in a gin and tonic can instantly transport you to sunnier stress-free climes and lemon water brought to the boil in a microwave can remove nasty food smells. Most crucially, though, it is the clever cook's third seasoning alongside salt and pepper – enhancing flavour and balancing taste. Make sure your fruit bowl is never without one.

DRINK

- Lemon barley water
- Lemon, root ginger, hot water & honey
- Lemonade
- Limoncello

GARNISH

- Wedges with fish
- Slices in drinks
- Candied peel
- Rind set in ice for drinks

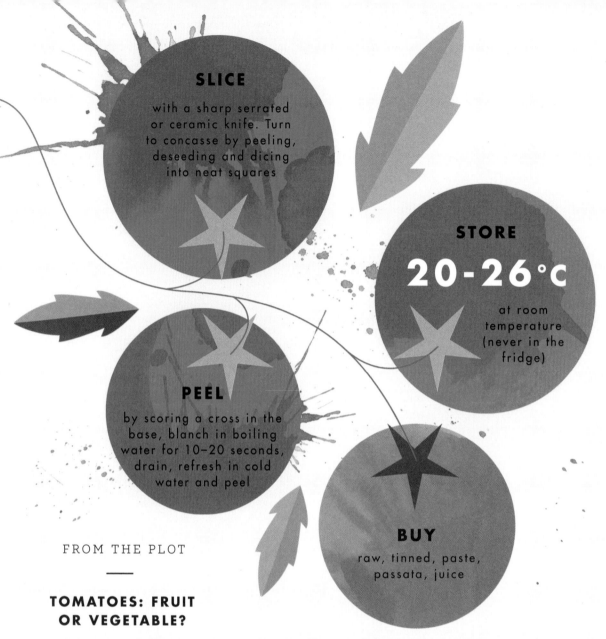

SLICE

with a sharp serrated or ceramic knife. Turn to concasse by peeling, deseeding and dicing into neat squares

STORE

20-26°C

at room temperature (never in the fridge)

PEEL

by scoring a cross in the base, blanch in boiling water for 10–20 seconds, drain, refresh in cold water and peel

BUY

raw, tinned, paste, passata, juice

FROM THE PLOT

—

TOMATOES: FRUIT OR VEGETABLE?

Given the fact this new kid on the culinary block only showed up on Mediterranean shores around the 16th century, it's testament to its incredible flavour and versatility that it's now considered the lifeblood of Italian cuisine.

Not a vegetable, although it's most certainly treated as such, this favoured fruit originated in the Americas and was brought over to Europe by the Spanish. It's related to the nightshade – and as such also aubergines, peppers and potatoes –

and now represents approximately 15% of the globe's vegetable production, making it a key player.

Indeed, many countries like to start and end their day with tomatoes. In northern Spain, the Catalonians rub toasted bread with garlic, tomatoes and olive oil for breakfast. Elsewhere – from Mexico with their huevos rancheros to Israel with their shakshuka – eggs are baked in a tomato sauce. It's a favourite in soups; think warming cream of tomato, right through

to chilled gazpacho. Tomatoes can even be drunk – as in the classic 1920s Parisian cocktail, Bloody Mary, which sees tomato juice, vodka, salt, pepper and Worcestershire sauce combined. (Try a contemporary variation with grated fresh wasabi and lime.)

The tomato's most famous outing though, has to be in a classic Italian sauce where, at its most basic, tomatoes are stewed and reduced with garlic and herbs and used to dress pasta or top a pizza.

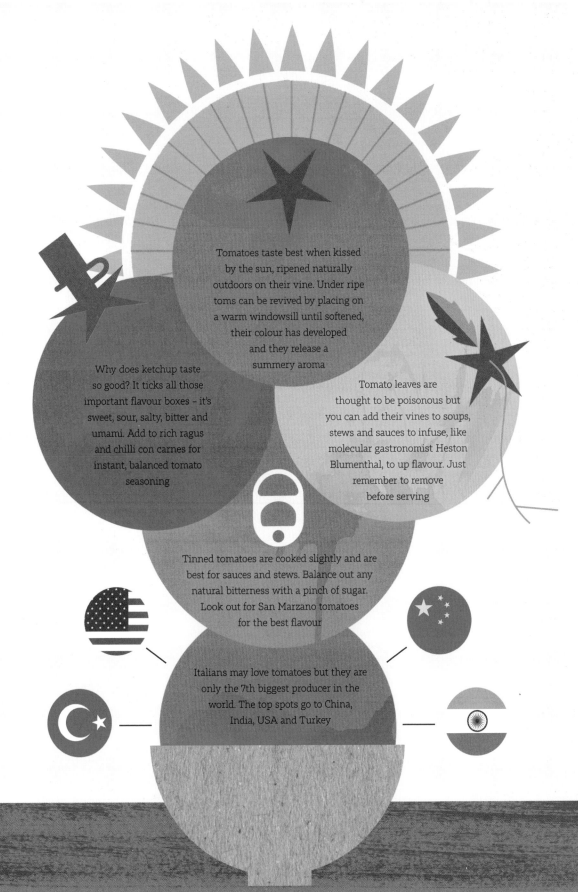

Tomatoes taste best when kissed by the sun, ripened naturally outdoors on their vine. Under ripe toms can be revived by placing on a warm windowsill until softened, their colour has developed and they release a summery aroma

Why does ketchup taste so good? It ticks all those important flavour boxes – it's sweet, sour, salty, bitter and umami. Add to rich ragus and chilli con carnes for instant, balanced tomato seasoning

Tomato leaves are thought to be poisonous but you can add their vines to soups, stews and sauces to infuse, like molecular gastronomist Heston Blumenthal, to up flavour. Just remember to remove before serving

Tinned tomatoes are cooked slightly and are best for sauces and stews. Balance out any natural bitterness with a pinch of sugar. Look out for San Marzano tomatoes for the best flavour

Italians may love tomatoes but they are only the 7th biggest producer in the world. The top spots go to China, India, USA and Turkey

Avocado leaves are often used in Mexican dishes for their anise flavour

Mexico is the biggest producer and exporter of avocados

12.5% more potassium per gram than a banana

19
K

1 avocado tree can produce up to

500

fruits a year

Also known as alligator pears (thanks to their knobbly green skin) and butter fruit (thanks to their super-smooth flesh)

Ripe avocados should yield slightly when pressed but have no sunken spots or blemishes

OTHER

HASS

80%
of the world's cultivated avocados are Hass, a modern Mexican-Guatemalan hybrid

3
'RACES' OF AVOCADO

MEXICAN
Richest in oil with leaves that smell like anise – best for sauces and dips

GUATEMALAN
Round fruits with rough and thick skin

WEST INDIAN
Produce the largest fruits, with a slight sweetness and much less oil – best for salads

---

AVOCADO: THE ALLIGATOR PEAR

Walk down the street in Colombia and for every 100 people you'll find five men selling ripe fuerte avocados by the cartload. Here they eat this fruit (yes, fruit – it's from the Lauraceae family, making it botanical cousins with cinnamon and bay) with everything from rice and meat, to chips and salad, or sliced into a sandwich.

There are three original races of the avocado and now 100s of hybrids in a variety of shapes (from round and fat, like an apple, to thin and bell-bottomed, like a pear), sizes (think plum to human head) and colours (ranging from yellowy-green, to purple and black).

Its creamy blandness is best kept simple (lime, salt and chilli being its best friends) and is better raw than cooked as it can turn bitter. The most famous avocado dish of them all is the Mexican dip, guacamole, but this fruit is also the superhero of brunches – my current go-to is grilled cheese on an English muffin, topped with slices of fried chorizo, creamy hass avocado, a poached egg and lashings of Sriracha – and champion of lunches. It's packed with fibre (more so than most fruits), potassium, vitamins C, E and K, and has almost double the 'good' monounsaturated fats of fresh salmon. Basically, it's an all-round good egg.

CUT

TWIST

SLICE & SCOOP

GO SAVOURY!

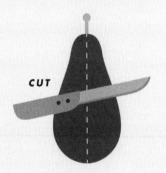

California roll
(Inside-out sushi with crab, cucumber and avocado)

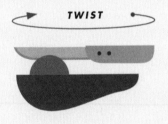

Guacamole
(Dip with chilli, coriander, lime and tomato)

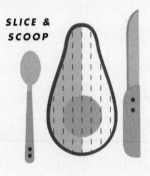

Chilled soup
(Particularly good with cucumber, tangy yoghurt or buttermilk, and dill)

GO SWEET!

Jus alpukat
(Indonesian chilled sweet drink with milk, sometimes coffee, and chocolate syrup)

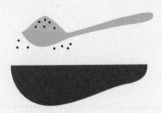

Sprinkle with sugar
(A Brazilian favourite)

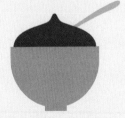

Chocolate mousse
(Popular with the raw food crowd – swap dairy for avos and blend with raw cacao or cocoa powder)

TYPES OF PEPPERS	SCOVILLE HEAT UNITS
PURE CAPSAICIN	16,000,000
POLICE PEPPER SPRAY	5,300,000
CAROLINA REAPER	1,569,300
TRINIDAD SCORPION	1,463,700
BHUT JOLOKIA	1,041,427
DORSET NAGA	923,000
RED SAVINA HABANERO	250,000-577,000
CHOCOLATE HABANERO	200,000-385,000
SCOTCH BONNET	150,000-325,000
ORANGE HABANERO	150,000-325,000
FATALI	125,000-325,000
DEVIL'S TONGUE	125,000-325,000
KUMATAKA	125,000-150,000
DATIL	100,000-300,000
BIRD'S EYE	100,000-225,000
JAMAICAN HOT	100,000-200,000
BOHEMIAN	95,000-115,000
TABICHE	85,000-115,000
TEPIN	80,000-240,000
HAIMEN	70,000-80,000
CHILTEPIN	60,000-85,000
THAI	50,000-100,000
YATSUFUSA	50,000-75,000
PEQUIN	40,000-58,000
SUPER CHILE	40,000-50,000
SANTAKA	40,000-50,000
CAYENNE	30,000-50,000
TABASCO	30,000-50,000
AJI	30,000-50,000
JALORO	30,000-50,000
DE ARBOL	15,000-30,000
MANZANO	12,000-30,000
HIDALGO	6,000-10,000
PUYA	5,000-10,000
HOT WAX	5,000-10,000
CHIPOTLE	5,000-8,000
JALAPEÑO	2,500-8,000
GUAJILLO	2,500-5,000
MIRASOL	2,500-5,000
ROCOTILLO	1,500-2,500
PASILLA	1,000-2,000
MULATO	1,000-2,000
ANCHO	1,000-2,000
POBLANO	1,000-2,000
ESPANOLA	1,000-2,000
PULLA	700-3,000
CORONADO	700-1,000
NUMEX BIG JIM	500-2,500
SANGRIA	500-2,500
ANAHEIM	500-2,500
SANTA FE GRANDE	500-750
EL PASO	500-700
PEPPERONCINI	100-500
CHERRY	0-500
PIMENTO	0
BELL PEPPER	0

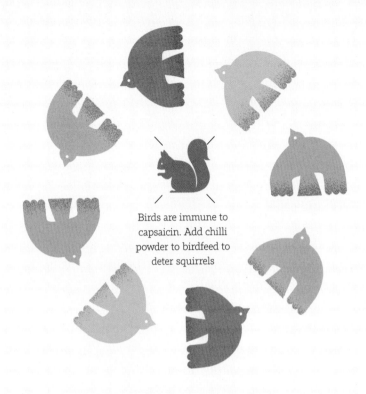

Birds are immune to capsaicin. Add chilli powder to birdfeed to deter squirrels

—

CHILLIES: HOT STUFF

Few foods can have such an impact on our palates, with so little calorific effect, as the chilli pepper. Cultivated for thousands of years and brought over to Europe by Christopher Columbus, the chilli is an integral component of many cuisines and cultures around the world – the fruity heat in the Caribbean's jerk chicken, the smoky prickle in a Mexican mole poblano, or the vibrant, sweet red kick of paprika in a Spanish chorizo.

But a chilli isn't just a chilli, of course. They come in all manner of shapes (bells and bonnets, to witches' fingers and friars' hats); textures (smooth or wrinkled); colours (red, yellow and green, right through to purple, black and brown); and, perhaps most notably, heats (from the gentle lip tingle of jalapeño to the entire-mouth burn of a Dorset naga).

In fact, they can be broken down into five main types. Annuum is the most widely cultivated and includes some of the most well-known chilli varieties – think cayenne, bell pepper, jalapeño, pimento and paprika. They'll have single (often white, or white with a purple tinge) flowers along their stem. Chinense chillies are some of the hottest

around – Scotch bonnet, red savino and habanero, to name a few – although there is the odd mild wild card such as the Trinidad perfume. Both, though, are characterized by a distinctly fruity, almost apricot-like, aroma, and often lantern-like, small, round shape.

Baccatum are distinguished by brown or green spots on the petals of their flowers, as well as their uniquely shaped and often wrinkled fruits; while frutescens, popular in African cooking, tend to be straight and small, most famously the Tabasco, piri piri and bird's eye. Pubescens are the least cultivated and denoted by their black seeds, hairy leaves and thick-skinned flesh. These chillies can grow to the size of small apples given half the chance.

Every chilli, though, contains capsaicin – the bit that makes it hot. In 1912, American pharmacist Wilbur Scoville developed the Scoville Heat Unit (SHU) scale through dilution of the chilli into sugar syrup, with a human taste panel. Nowadays, though, a more accurate method called High-Performance Liquid Chromatography (HPLC) is used to scientifically record the burn.

COURGETTE: THE GARDENER'S FRIEND

If herbs on the kitchen windowsill are the baby steps into growing your own veg, then courgettes are the stabilizers on your first bike. They take some care to grow but can pretty much be left to their own devices once the first tender shoots poke through the soil. And once they start growing , boy, they just don't stop.

Close cousins with cucumber, like pumpkins, and melons, the courgettes we see on our plates today were most likely developed in Italy and have only really been eaten with any gusto elsewhere, particularly in the UK or USA, in the last century.

They come yellow, green or striped; can be eaten young, when they are barely 8cm long, but are best at around 20cm. Any bigger and they'll become watery and that delicate taste will turn plain bland.

They love Mediterranean flavours (tomato, garlic, onion and lemon) and floral herbs (basil, oregano and thyme) and are a great sponge for spice – the ultimate filler to any meal. Use them in curries, slice them into stir-fries, or bathe in garlicky butter. Just never, ever boil them and avoid overcooking where possible.

Keep the crunch!

The golden flowers are edible too, but if you want your courgette to keep growing only pick the male flowers attached to the stalks, rather than the vegetable itself. Stuff with a combination of 250g ricotta, 75g grated strong hard cheese, the zest of 1 lemon and 1 tbsp lemon juice, 1 tbsp dried chilli flakes and a handful of fresh parsley and mint, finely chopped. Dip in a batter (double cream consistency) of 150g self-raising flour, 50g cornflour and 250ml ice-cold soda water and deep-fry in vegetable oil at 180°C until golden and puffy all over. Drain and enjoy hot.

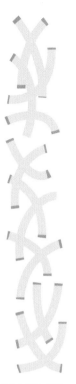
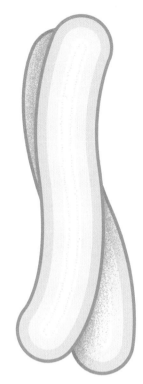
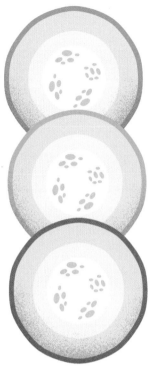
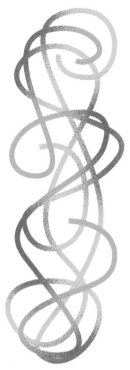

GRATE ME

Make a thick savoury pancake batter and add grated courgette, finely chopped fresh mint and crumbled Feta. Shallow fry in olive or rapeseed oil and serve with Greek yoghurt

PEEL ME

Peel raw courgettes into long ribbons and combine with shavings of Grana Padano, halved cherry tomatoes, torn fresh basil leaves, sliced red chilli, lemon juice and coriander-leaf-infused olive or rapeseed oil

SLICE ME

Layer a baking dish with slices of courgettes, tomatoes, red onion, garlic, olive oil, fresh thyme and grated Cheddar and bake in a hot oven until soft and caramelized

SPIRALIZE ME

Use a spiralizer, or julienne using a knife, to create long strands of raw 'courgetti'. Dress with fresh basil pesto or romesco sauce

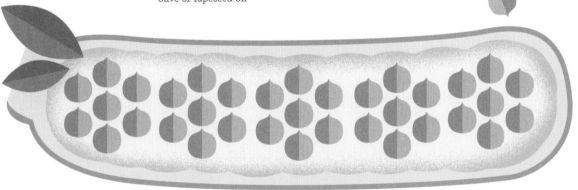

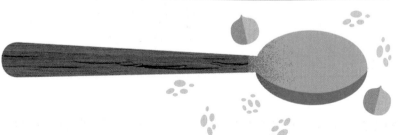

STUFF ME

Scoop out the seeds of larger/ overgrown courgettes and stuff with cooked minced pork (or chickpeas for a veggie version) seasoned with ras el hanout and bake in a medium-hot oven until tender

If you don't like
it greasy, try
brushing slices with
oil and grilling or
baking rather
than frying

Pea aubergines
are best in Asian
curries

OLIVE OIL AND
AUBERGINES ARE BFFS

Once cooked, the spongy flesh of an
aubergine becomes naturally creamy,
silky and smooth, making it perfect
for dips and popular with vegans, as
no animal fats are required! Various
aubergine 'caviars' exist but the most
famous is the Levantine baba ganoush.
Roast whole over hot coals on the
barbecue, or a gas flame, to add a smoky
flavour, scoop out the flesh and mash
together with minced garlic. Season
with lemon juice, salt and pepper. You
can also add tahini, Greek yoghurt,
labneh and olive oil, or make like the
Colombians who mash aubergine
together with plantain in boronía
barranquillera, or the Serbians who
combine theirs with roasted red
peppers to make ajvar.

Aubergines love tang!
Try with buttermilk,
miso, sheep's
cheese, tamarind
or yoghurt

The long,
thin Japanese
and Chinese
aubergines
have fewer
seeds, tend
to be less
bitter than
their bulbous
counterparts,
and are best in
stir-fries.

Italy likes theirs baked in melanzane Parmigiana with a rich tomato sauce, stringy mozzarella and sharp Parmesan cheese.

Spain likes to fry theirs in slices for tapas.

Greece likes theirs sliced, layered and baked with minced meat, cinnamon and a creamy, egg-enriched béchamel sauce in a moussaka.

AUBERGINE: EGGPLANT

Bred from the wild nightshade like the tomato, pepper and potato the aubergine in all its black, purple, white and green varieties is actually a berry, not a vegetable.

Like the best of us, aubergines get bitter and wrinkly with age and are best when young and fresh. Look for a heavy fruit, with firm, taut, glossy skin with no blemishes, and cut just before cooking otherwise the creamy flesh will discolour.

Traditional recipes call for 'degorging' where the aubergines are salted, rinsed and drained before cooking to remove bitterness, but it's really not necessary with modern strains. Some say that salting also helps aubergines absorb less fat during cooking but as long as you choose the right fruit for the job, I don't think this is necessary either.

Patience is a virtue from the cooking to the eating. Never undercook and always serve warm, not hot, for the best flavour.

Aubergines are prized in Turkish cuisine and one of the most celebrated dishes is stuffed aubergines called imam bayildi, which translates as 'the imam fainted'. Rumours clash over whether it was the taste or the cost of the olive oil in the dish that caused him to swoon, but regardless it's a delicious combo of caramelized onions, garlic, tomatoes, parsley and olive oil, served at room temperature.

Various aubergine stews exist – its flesh acting like a flavour sponge for whatever it's partnered with – from Provençal's ratatouille and Spain's pisto, to North India's bharta, Sicily's sweet and sour caponata, or Sichuan's fish-fragrant dish with minced pork.

Prick aubergines before roasting them whole in the oven to stop them exploding

CABBAGE: BRASSICA BASICS

Shredded into American slaw, packed with salt in German sauerkraut, or rolled and stuffed with minced pork like the Romanians do, cabbages are loved around the world. But they are also hated, too, and that would be thanks to dimethyl sulphide.

It's a chemical compound that has a pokey smell (an aroma that haunts many a British school hall), which only gets worse the longer the cabbage is cooked. The key to cooking this most ancient of brassicas – and to keep the smell to a minimum – is to keep it quick. Instead of long boiling; steam or steam-fry (with a small amount of water in the bottom of a frying pan or wok), or even stir-fry with oil, which will add a nutty, caramelized flavour.

The original wild cabbage was more like kale and it's been valued since the ancient Egyptians, Romans and Greeks for its health properties and even as a preventative cure for getting drunk. Now various incarnations of the cabbage are available around the globe – red (or really, a deep purple), white and various shades of green; some round, others conical; some with heads, others stalks with leafy greens. Whichever you choose, preparation and cooking is easy. Simply remove any tough or limp outer leaves and slice, grate or roll as required, cook and enjoy.

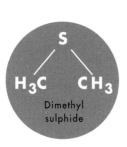

Dimethyl sulphide

This chemical compound can also be found in asparagus, beetroot, truffle and seafood, and is particularly noticeable if you cook cabbage for a long time

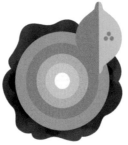

Keep your red cabbage purple with an acid (such as citrus juice or vinegar) while cooking, otherwise it will turn blue

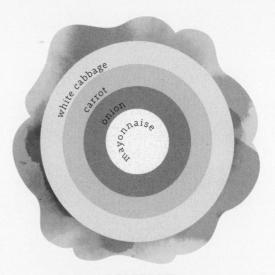

white cabbage
carrot
onion
mayonnaise

COLESLAW

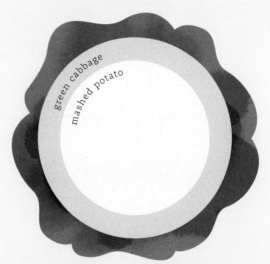

green cabbage
mashed potato

COLCANNON

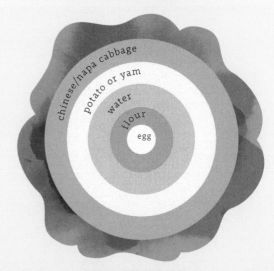

chinese/napa cabbage
potato or yam
water
flour
egg

OKONOMIYAKI
(Savoury pancake)

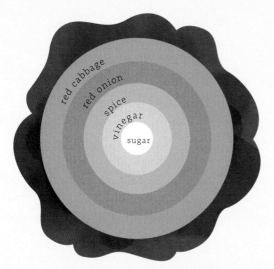

BRAISED RED CABBAGE

red cabbage
red onion
spice
vinegar
sugar

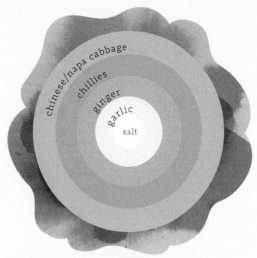

KIMCHI

chinese/napa cabbage
chillies
ginger
garlic
salt

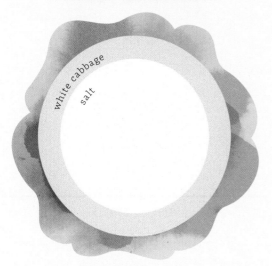

SAUERKRAUT

white cabbage
salt

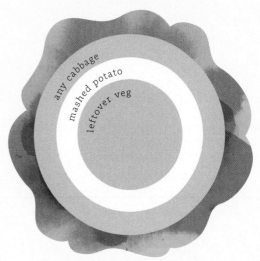

BUBBLE & SQUEAK

any cabbage
mashed potato
leftover veg

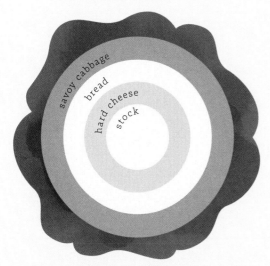

ITALIAN BREAD & CABBAGE SOUP

savoy cabbage
bread
hard cheese
stock

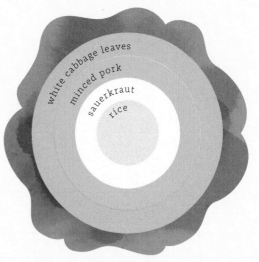

SARMALE
(Stuffed cabbage)

white cabbage leaves
minced pork
sauerkraut
rice

29

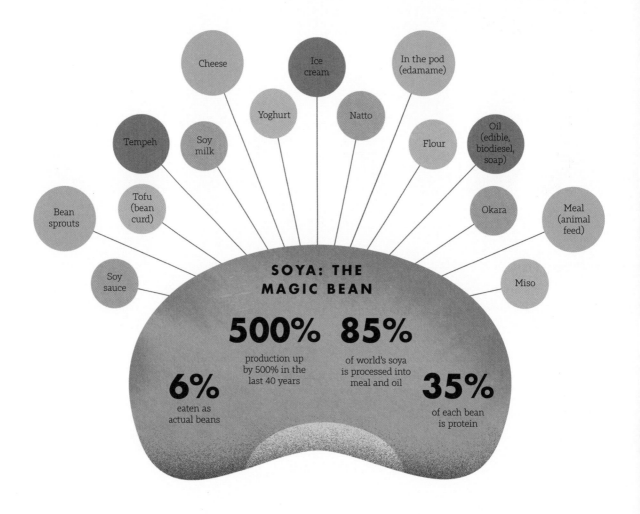

Cheese

Ice cream

In the pod (edamame)

Yoghurt

Natto

Tempeh

Soy milk

Flour

Oil (edible, biodiesel, soap)

Bean sprouts

Tofu (bean curd)

Okara

Meal (animal feed)

Soy sauce

Miso

SOYA: THE MAGIC BEAN

500%
production up by 500% in the last 40 years

85%
of world's soya is processed into meal and oil

6%
eaten as actual beans

35%
of each bean is protein

FROM THE PLOT

—

BEANS: FULL OF 'EM

Whether you like yours white, soft and stewed, and swimming in tomato sauce straight from the tin, or green in the pod, blanched and served up with tuna, olives and sliced eggs in a Niçoise salad, beans are one of the best foods you can eat. (And not just for their flavour.)

While the majority of beans are indigenous to the Americas, it is China's soya bean that is the most globally significant. As a 'complete'

protein (with all eight amino acids essential for our health), it is incredibly nutritious and now the most widely cultivated legume worldwide. They can be eaten in their pod like the Japanese do, where they are called edamame; on their own; sprouting; or even as tofu. But, they definitely aren't the best tasting. For that, you'll have to look back across the Pacific.

Broad or fava beans (even if Pythagoras – you know, the maths guy

– didn't like them) have long been the favourite bean of Europeans and beyond. Snuggled in their protective, fluffy sleeping bag-like pod, they can be eaten young and raw, blanched in salads, dried as a salty snack or stewed with spices and mashed like the Egyptians do for their national breakfast dish, ful medames. If you're eating them fresh, just be sure to double pod the beans, to remove the tough waxy skins.

Haricot (navy) beans

Small, creamy and the star of tinned baked beans.
A sponge for flavour so great in soups and stews

Broad (fava) beans

Medium, green and best double-podded. Delicious
raw, blanched or dried. Toss young beans with
creamy goat's cheese, caraway seeds and mint

Black-eyed peas

One half of Jamaica's rice and peas and essential
to the southern United States' hoppin' John, with
fatty cuts of pork and rice

French (snap) beans

Green and eaten in the pod. Light blanch or boil is all that's
required. Best in cold, warm or hot salads. Beware of the squeak

Butter beans

Large, creamy and soft. Loves garlic
and woody herbs. Great mashed as an
alternative to potato or as a vegetarian dip

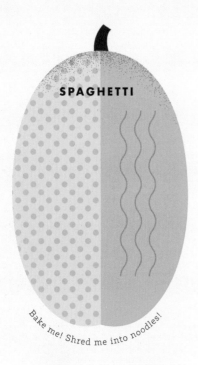

SPAGHETTI

Bake me! Shred me into noodles!

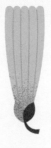

PUMPKIN: PATCH TO PIE

The symbol of a season on the turn, a tool to ward off evil spirits and the fodder of fairytales – pumpkins are probably the most famous of all the winter squash but are they the most delicious? Related to cucumbers, courgettes and melons – and technically a fruit – these hardy squash come in a spectrum of shapes, sizes and colours, from dusky blues and creamy yellows to egg-yolk orange and moss green. Pumpkins, which are native to America, are best known for their part in the Thanksgiving tradition of the same continent (puréed with warming winter spices, as the filling for a sweet pie) or disemboweled and carved for Halloween. They can be brewed into beer, grated into cakes, or simply mashed with butter – even the leaves and seeds can be eaten. But would you recognize the right squash for the job?

Toast seeds with salt or soy sauce and spice for a tasty snack!

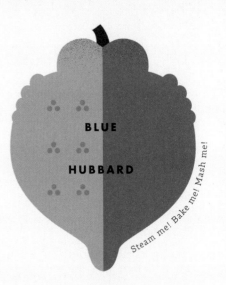

BLUE

HUBBARD

Steam me! Bake me! Mash me!

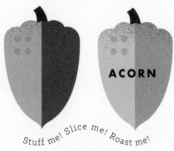

ACORN

Stuff me! Slice me! Roast me!

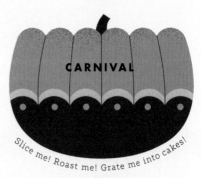

CARNIVAL

Slice me! Roast me! Grate me into cakes!

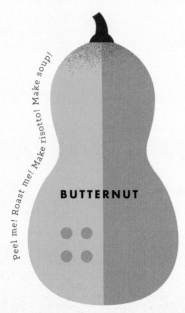

Peel me! Roast me! Make risotto! Make soup!

BUTTERNUT

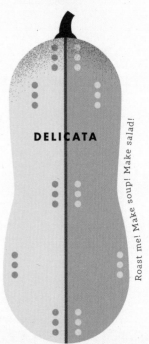

DELICATA

Roast me! Make soup! Make salad!

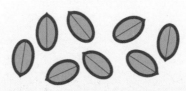

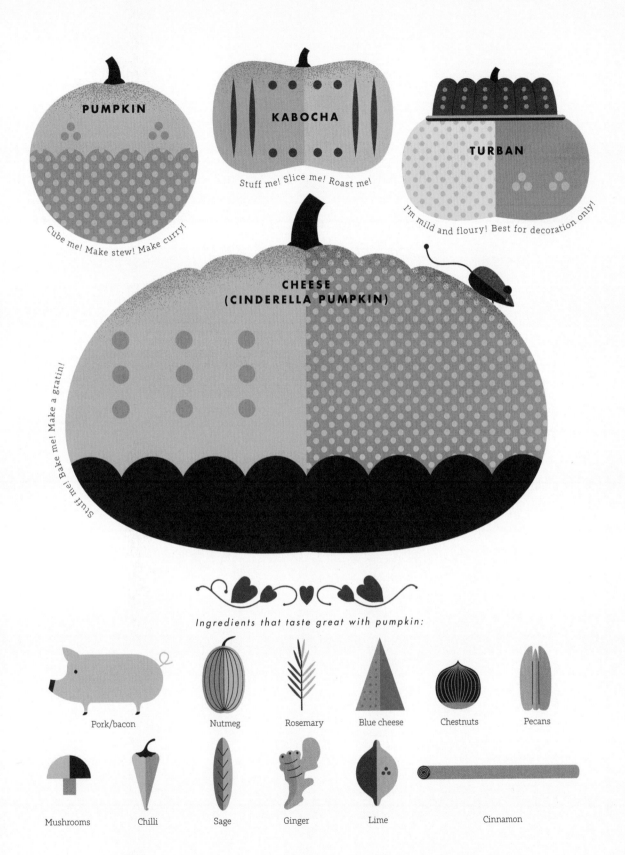

PUMPKIN

Cube me! Make stew! Make curry!

KABOCHA

Stuff me! Slice me! Roast me!

TURBAN

I'm mild and floury! Best for decoration only!

**CHEESE
(CINDERELLA PUMPKIN)**

Stuff me! Bake me! Make a gratin!

Ingredients that taste great with pumpkin:

Pork/bacon

Nutmeg

Rosemary

Blue cheese

Chestnuts

Pecans

Mushrooms

Chilli

Sage

Ginger

Lime

Cinnamon

BEET: IT

As attention-seeking vegetables go, beetroot's a real try hard. A descendant of wild sea beet, which can still be found on coastlines across Europe through to Asia, modern beetroot varieties can be eaten root to top and come in shades from shocking crimson to golden yellow and even white and pink stripes.

Eastern Europeans love the magenta globe roots and use them to make the region's most famous soup – borscht – that can be served hot or cold, clear or creamy. The beet is also well known for getting pickled – the Lebanese use it alongside turnips, making them blush, while the British traditionally drown slices of boiled beet in harsh malt vinegar.

But it's not just flashy colour or its distinctive earthy sweet flavour that makes beetroot a winner. It's seriously good for you, too. The Romans recognized its medicinal properties first and it's still hailed now as a modern 'superfood' with its powerful antioxidants and vitamins. Boil it, bake it, grate it, roast it, fry it or slice it thin – everything looks rosy with beetroot.

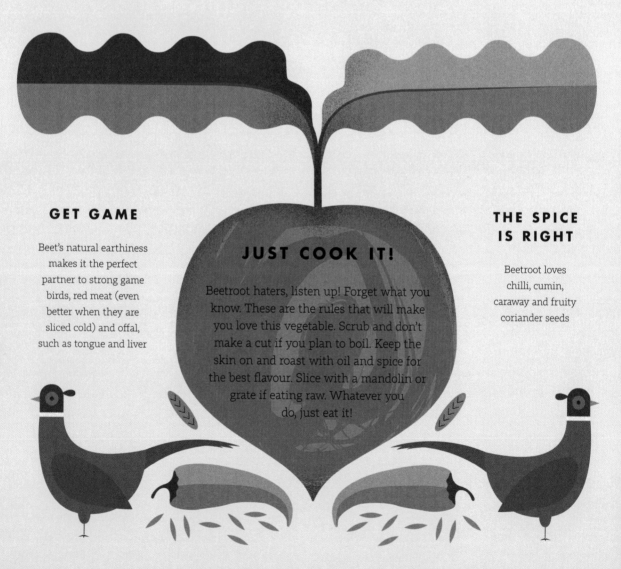

GET GAME

Beet's natural earthiness makes it the perfect partner to strong game birds, red meat (even better when they are sliced cold) and offal, such as tongue and liver

JUST COOK IT!

Beetroot haters, listen up! Forget what you know. These are the rules that will make you love this vegetable. Scrub and don't make a cut if you plan to boil. Keep the skin on and roast with oil and spice for the best flavour. Slice with a mandolin or grate if eating raw. Whatever you do, just eat it!

THE SPICE IS RIGHT

Beetroot loves chilli, cumin, caraway and fruity coriander seeds

TRY ADDING TANG

No beetroot salad is complete nowadays without a crumble of goat's cheese but the truth is it will happily share its plate with anything with a tang – labneh, sour cream, crème fraîche, buttermilk, gherkins, orange segments or even fresh apple. It does love vinegar, too, but swap malt for sherry, red wine or balsamic vinegar in moderation

EATS SHOOTS AND LEAVES

Picked fresh, beetroot leaves are edible, too. Treat like spinach – washed young leaves can be used in salad, more mature should be quickly sautéed

BAKE IT TILL YOU MAKE IT

Who doesn't love carrot cake? It makes sense that similarly sweet beetroot should work then, right? Many bakers agree, mixing beetroot into chocolate cake/brownie/muffin mixes but it does add earthiness. I'll take a savoury muffin instead, thanks

STICK TO YOUR ROOTS

Like many vegetables, beetroot likes those that it shares ground with. Pair with other sweet root veg, like carrots and parsnips, and woody herbs like rosemary and thyme, or soft dill. It also loves fiery horseradish in relishes, salads and soups

GO FISH

In Scandinavia and Baltic countries they love their beetroot and oily fish – think herring, mackerel and salmon. Add beetroot to any fish cure (or indeed anything – from gnocchi to pasta and bread) and it will impart its pretty purple colour, too

—

ASPARAGUS: BRIT SPEARS

The ancient Greeks first cottoned on to just how ace asparagus really is. Fast and easy to cook, and packed with goodies (from vitamins A, C and E, to fibre and folic acid), it's little surprise that festivals dedicated to the spears are celebrated around the world.

China is the biggest producer (and consumer) of the stuff (some 20x more than the next grower, Peru) but it is perhaps most revered in Europe. Grown in sandy soil from a 'crown', it can take three years to produce the first harvest and, once it reaches delicious maturity, needs to be hand cut, so precious are those delicate stalks.

An example of that most mystical of taste sensations 'umami', the singular flavour of asparagus (green, purple, white or wild) is best treated simply. Eat in season (it usually straddles spring and summer) and fresh (it doesn't store well after being picked), ideally with some sort of tasty fat – whether that be a buttery hollandaise, a clean olive oil dressing and sharp, aged hard cheese, or a creamy pasta sauce punctuated with smoky lardons of bacon and topped with a rubble of golden breadcrumbs.

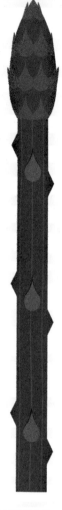

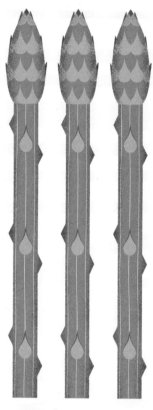

GREEN

A favourite of the Brits and widely eaten across the US, Australasia and China, these thick, tall stems should have tight tips and need only be prepared by gently bending to find the natural snapping point to remove the tough base. Steam, boil, blanch or grill; barbecue, roast, stir-fry or sauté. Whatever you do, keep it quick. Overcook and you'll lose the natural sweetness

PURPLE

The clever Italians created this variety. These spears have less fibre and tend to be sweeter. Snap and peel raw into pretty edible ribbons for salads

WHAT PAIRS WELL WITH ASPARAGUS?

Hazelnuts

Cheese

Soy sauce

Anchovies

Eggs

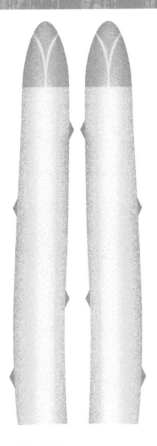

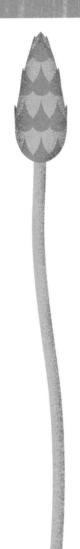

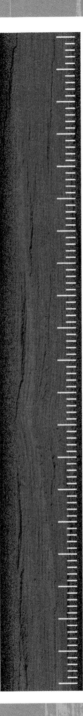

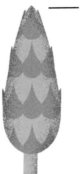

24 HOURS

HOW BIG?

Asparagus spears can
grow 25cm in 24 hours
in the right conditions

WHITE

Prized in Germany and across
much of central Europe, these
stalks are the same as green
asparagus but have been
deprived of light (either by
burying them in soil or using
modern black polyhouses).
They're the problem child of the
family – tougher, so will need
snapping and peeling before
cooking, and bland – and are
prone to getting pickled

WILD

Where the wild asparagus
grows is a closely guarded
secret amongst greedy
foodies. Thin and delicious
eaten raw or blanched

Shallots

Peas

Smoked salmon

Lemon

Broad beans

Oyster sauce

GARLIC: ALL-POWERFUL ALLIUM

You can buy it fresh or flaked, wet or wild, powdered or as paste; however you consider it, garlic is a titan of the allium world. It's a punchy and fiery smack of flavour when eaten raw, and a sweet and mellow culinary hug when roasted. It gets around too – few ingredients feature so heavily in so many cuisines around the world.

The one party the popular garlic will never be welcome at, though, is a sweet one. Salted caramel? Delicious. Carrot cake? Top notch. Bacon brownies? Okay, sort of get it. Garlic custard? Get out of town! Make sure you know which garlic to use, when and how, with these ultimate garlic lifehacks.

PICK ME!

There are hundreds of types of garlic but they broadly fit into two main categories: softnecks, which are easy to grow and the most commonly available, and hardnecks, which have the best flavour

DON'T BE BITTER!

Garlic that has a green shoot at its heart will be bitter and particularly pungent – remove!

STORE ME!

Keep garlic bulbs together (separated cloves dry out quicker) in a cool, dry environment for 2-3 weeks

A cold, damp fridge is too similar to the ground and will cause the garlic to shoot

Wet or wild garlic should be kept in the fridge for no more than a week

GO WILD!

For a mild garlic flavour, raw or cooked, look out for young, fresh garlic bulbs also known as 'wet garlic', or its cousin 'bear garlic', which grows wild in shaded woodland. Blitz the flat green leaves into pesto or shred into risottos and omelettes

COOK ME!

Want to transform harsh, hot garlic to sticky and sweet garlic? Just slice off the top of a whole bulb, drizzle in olive oil, wrap in foil and roast for 30–40 minutes at 200°C

ATTACK ME!

For a milder flavour, use a knife to slice and dice, while garlic purée will taste stronger and can be made by applying pressure with the blade and salt, or with a pestle and mortar.

PEEL ME!

Forget the fancy gadgets, bring out the most useful tool in the kitchen – your hand. Apply pressure to the garlic bulb with the heel of your hand to release the cloves, then do the same to the clove to release the papery husk

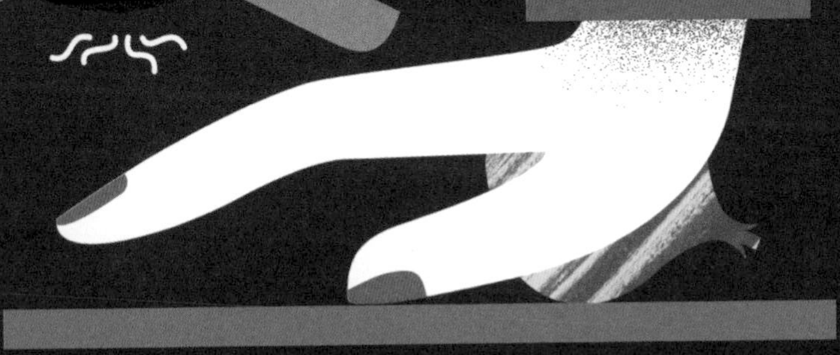

THE BEST THINGS IN LIFE ARE 3

Garlic is the base of some of the world's best threesomes:

Garlic Chilli Ginger

Garlic Egg yolks Olive oil

Garlic Basil Tomato

Garlic Butter Bread

Garlic Onion Celery

Garlic Rosemary Lamb

39

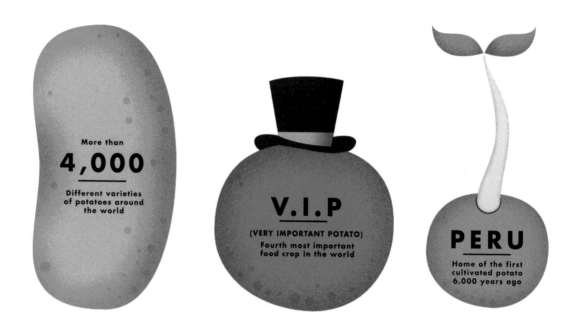

More than
4,000
Different varieties
of potatoes around
the world

V.I.P
(VERY IMPORTANT POTATO)
Fourth most important
food crop in the world

PERU
Home of the first
cultivated potato
6,000 years ago

—

POTATO: SPUD YOU LIKE

As the world's fourth most important crop (behind maize, wheat and rice), it seems a disservice to this humble tuber to call it simply a spud. The potato has thousands of varieties around the world, the majority of which can be found in its country of origin, Peru, where the Incas first cultivated it some 6,000 years ago. They come in all shapes, sizes, colours and textures, and should be chosen according to their destined dish.

'Early' and 'Second Early' varieties might also be known as 'new potatoes' and are usually waxy, smaller, good boiled or steamed for salads, and roasted whole in their skins (where all the fibre and much of the nutrients are contained) with a drizzle of olive oil, sea salt and a sprinkling of hot, smoked paprika. Available in late spring/early summer, Anya, Maris Peer, Pink Fir Apple and Charlotte are particular favourites – the latter being especially good sliced thinly on a mandolin and baked with cream and garlic and topped with a strong, hard cheese like an aged Pecorino Romano. In the UK, foodies hungrily await the Jersey Royal season, these tiny tubers are grown just off the southern coast on the island of

Jersey between March and July, and have a distinctive sweet, summery flavour.

'Main crop' potatoes, harvested in autumn, are larger, dry and floury, making them perfect for roasting, baking in their skins and deep-frying in fat for glorious thick-cut chips or skinny fries. Maris Piper is probably the most famous potato of this ilk and certainly the most consumed across Europe. In the UK alone, 19,000 hectares were dedicated to the crop in 2012. Their golden skin, creamy white flesh and fluffy texture make them perfect for everything from oven-baked wedges to creamy mash.

For the best lump-free mash though, look to smooth potatoes, like the firm, red-skinned Desiree, which should be peeled then boiled until soft, drained and placed back on the hob to dry, before being pressed through a ricer. The key is then to beat the potato with butter and whole milk, and plenty of salt and pepper. Mashed potato is great as a base for other dishes, too; as a meat or fish pie topping, combined with flour and egg for Italian gnocchi, shallow fried with leftover vegetables for British bubble 'n' squeak, or combined with the day's catch to make it go further in a fishcake.

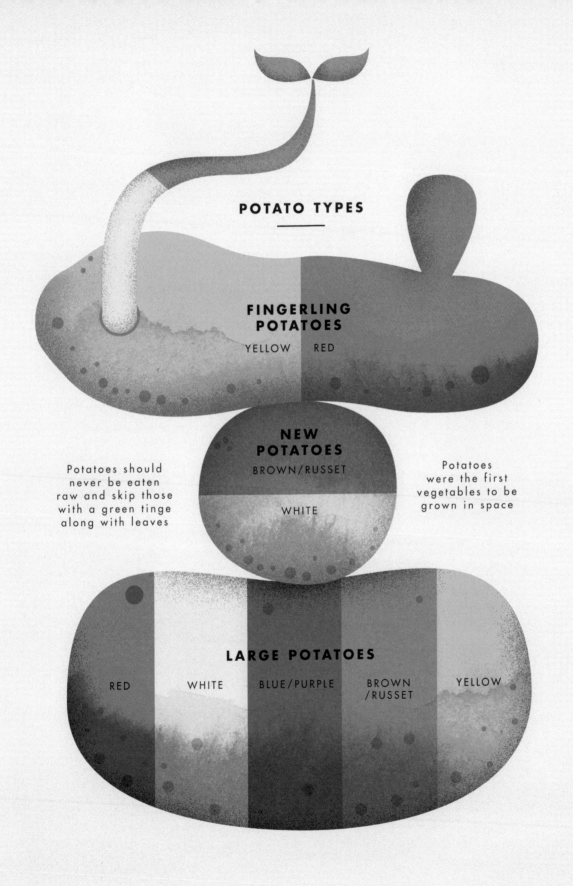

POTATO TYPES

FINGERLING POTATOES

YELLOW   RED

NEW POTATOES

BROWN/RUSSET

WHITE

Potatoes should never be eaten raw and skip those with a green tinge along with leaves

Potatoes were the first vegetables to be grown in space

LARGE POTATOES

RED   WHITE   BLUE/PURPLE   BROWN /RUSSET   YELLOW

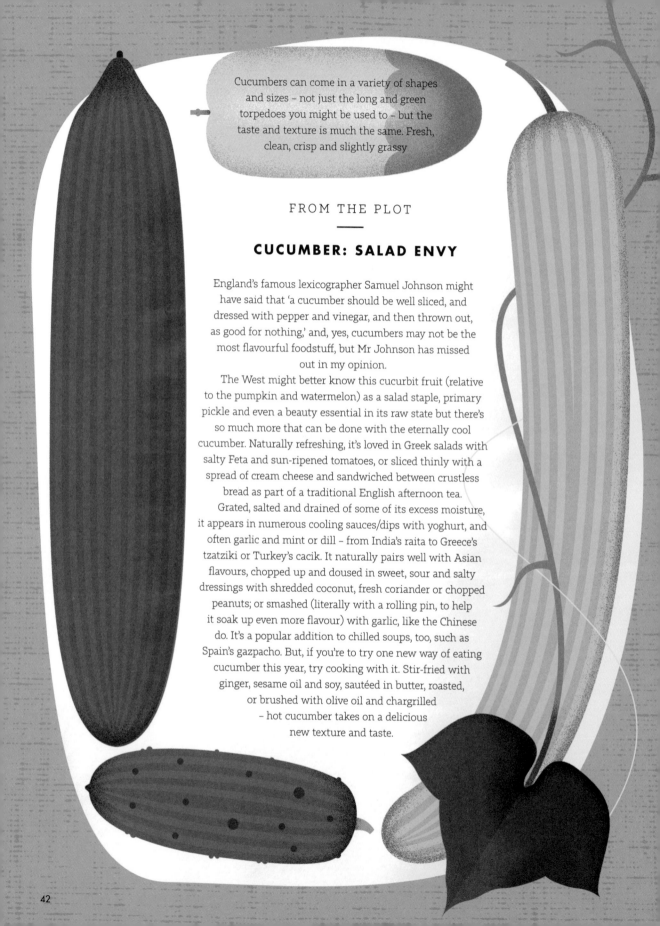

Cucumbers can come in a variety of shapes and sizes – not just the long and green torpedoes you might be used to – but the taste and texture is much the same. Fresh, clean, crisp and slightly grassy

FROM THE PLOT

—

CUCUMBER: SALAD ENVY

England's famous lexicographer Samuel Johnson might have said that 'a cucumber should be well sliced, and dressed with pepper and vinegar, and then thrown out, as good for nothing,' and, yes, cucumbers may not be the most flavourful foodstuff, but Mr Johnson has missed out in my opinion.

The West might better know this cucurbit fruit (relative to the pumpkin and watermelon) as a salad staple, primary pickle and even a beauty essential in its raw state but there's so much more that can be done with the eternally cool cucumber. Naturally refreshing, it's loved in Greek salads with salty Feta and sun-ripened tomatoes, or sliced thinly with a spread of cream cheese and sandwiched between crustless bread as part of a traditional English afternoon tea. Grated, salted and drained of some of its excess moisture, it appears in numerous cooling sauces/dips with yoghurt, and often garlic and mint or dill – from India's raita to Greece's tzatziki or Turkey's cacik. It naturally pairs well with Asian flavours, chopped up and doused in sweet, sour and salty dressings with shredded coconut, fresh coriander or chopped peanuts; or smashed (literally with a rolling pin, to help it soak up even more flavour) with garlic, like the Chinese do. It's a popular addition to chilled soups, too, such as Spain's gazpacho. But, if you're to try one new way of eating cucumber this year, try cooking with it. Stir-fried with ginger, sesame oil and soy, sautéed in butter, roasted, or brushed with olive oil and chargrilled – hot cucumber takes on a delicious new texture and taste.

96% water

CUCUMBER IMPOSTERS

The leaves and purple flowers of the borage herb have a delicate cucumber flavour (freeze them into ice cubes or sprinkle over salads for a pretty garnish), while the so-called sea cucumber isn't even a cucumber at all – it's a marine animal and is considered a delicacy in parts of South East Asia

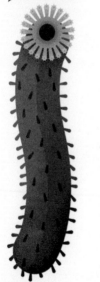

COOL AS A CUCUMBER

The inside of a cucumber is said to be around 6°C cooler than the outside air. That must be why slices of the stuff feel so soothing on puffy, sad eyes

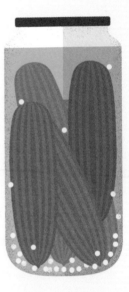

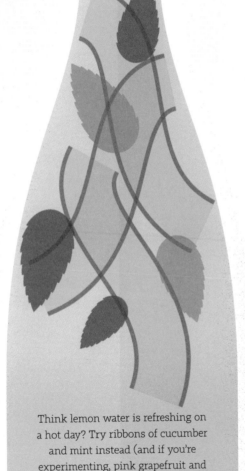

Think lemon water is refreshing on a hot day? Try ribbons of cucumber and mint instead (and if you're experimenting, pink grapefruit and crushed long or black pepper is rather good, too). Why not add it to some of your favourite cocktails, as well – from a simple G&T or a classic Pimms Cup with strawberries, to a minty Mojito or tequila- and lime-laced Margarita

IN A PICKLE

Small cucumbers are often jarred and pickled whole as gherkins and cornichons, but you can also slice larger cucumbers on a mandolin for delicious sweet and sour 'bread and butter' style pickles, or quickly pickle for fresh salads

Onions symbolized eternity to ancient Egyptians and they even buried them along with their pharaohs

Most of the volatile oil in an onion that can make you cry lies in the root. Chill the onion before chopping and leave the root until last to minimize the tears

Combine diced onion, carrot and celery in a mirepoix to form the base of many stocks, stews, sauces and soups

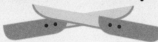

CHOP, CHOP!

How to slice and dice, minus the tears

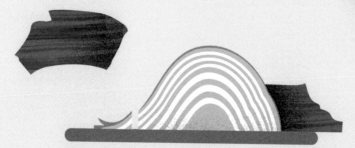

1 Start with a brown onion, large sharp knife and plastic chopping board. Slice in half (through the root and stem top).

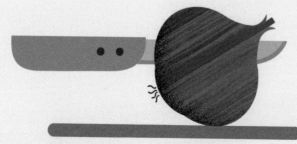

2 Chop off the stem top and peel away the brown skin leaving the root intact.

FROM THE PLOT

—

ONION: KNOW YOURS

The smell of onions caramelizing, ideally before being piled high on a hot dog, is something that few can resist. While rarely playing the lead in a dish, this humble allium thrives in its supporting role – adding layers of flavour and colour, and unrivalled depth, to dishes around the world.

While many varieties exist – indeed it is one of the world's

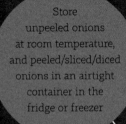

Store unpeeled onions at room temperature, and peeled/sliced/diced onions in an airtight container in the fridge or freezer

Stud whole onions with cloves and bay leaves to add aroma and depth to white sauces and when cooking Puy lentils

Don't buy into the caramelized onion myth – sticky, deeply golden onions can only be achieved by heating low and slow with oil and butter. Think 30 minutes up

Dry brown/yellow, white and red onions can last for months if stored correctly but discard any that have green shoots or are bruised

most popular crops to grow – it is the common dry brown/yellow, sweeter red and immature, milder spring onions (also known as scallions) that we use the most day to day. Raw, each variety has its own astringency and gentle heat, but if cooked with care and attention can be transformed into a sweet, mellow hum. Roast whole in their skins until soft and tender; slice and caramelize for a supremely cheap and satisfying French onion soup; or pep up mashed potato with flecks of green sliced spring onions like the Irish do in their champ.

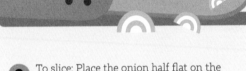

3 To slice: Place the onion half flat on the chopping board, holding the root with your fingers tucked in, and start slicing from the stem, working back to the root.

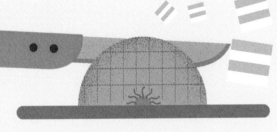

4 To dice: Place the onion half flat on the chopping board, holding the root with your fingers tucked in, turn and cut lengthways from stem to root every few mm but leave the root intact. Turn your knife and slice about 3x horizontally into the onion again leaving the root intact. Then slice down as before to produce fine dice.

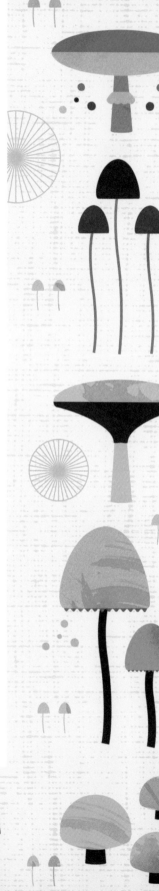

MUSHROOM: FOR FUNGI

Neither a vegetable nor an animal – the mushroom is one of nature's good guys, specifically, a fungi. Working in perfect symbiosis with their natural environment (whether that be shady woodland, open grassland or the cave-cum-nightclub-and-snail-farm that I once visited in the Loire, France), mushrooms are found and enjoyed in every continent. They were a symbol of immortality to the ancient Egyptians, they are an essential part of Chinese medicine and nowadays they're valued for being naturally low in fat and high in proteins and vitamins. But most importantly, they taste great, too.

They come in all manner of sizes and colours, ranging from white and brown, to yellow, orange, red, purple and even blue. Most have the familiar cap and stem – from the common white button mushroom to the revered cep – others have a skirt like the veiled lady, or even grow spines like North America's globular lion's mane. Their scents vary dramatically too – from aniseed or apricots, to carrot and coconut.

When it comes to edible mushrooms – the most popular being button, portobello, chanterelles, ceps, morels, oyster, shiitake and enoki – the trick is to cook them the right way. Never wash them (they're suckers for water), just lightly brush away the dirt. And unless eating them raw, sliced into a salad with dill and dressed with olive oil and lemon juice, most mushrooms are at their best when sautéed. The frying pan should be hot and with enough butter (for flavour) and oil (to stop the butter burning) to see the mushrooms (quartered or halved, don't slice) squeak and dance in the pan. Save the seasoning until their natural juices have evaporated and the fungi starts to caramelize and develop that addictive umami flavour. They are also great dried and used in stocks and risottos, or pickled in salads.

And what is earthy mushroom's best friend? Garlic, of course. But then again, who isn't a close acquaintance of this allium. Except, maybe, Dracula.

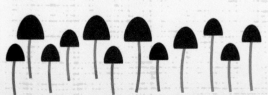

FUN(GI) FACTS

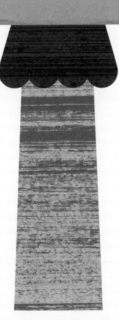

Mushrooms were once (and still can be) used to make natural dyes

A mushroom is 90% water

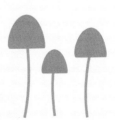

A devotee of mushrooms is called a mycophile

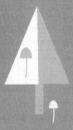

Mushrooms can grow on the ground, on trees and even in used coffee grounds

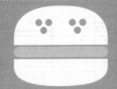

Mushrooms are often used as a meat replacement in burgers or Russia's classic beef stroganoff, thanks to its deep umami flavour. There's even a beefsteak fungus that looks like liver and 'bleeds' when cut

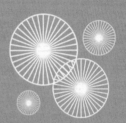

A mature mushroom can produce up to 16 billion spores

There are more than 70 bioluminescent (aka glow-in-the-dark) fungi although most are inedible. They provide a 'cold' light (often called fox or fairy fire) because they don't emit lots of heat, like a lightbulb, when illuminated

There are 1000s of different fungi and only a small percentage is safe to eat. Of those, even fewer are actually pleasant to eat. Some can cause hallucinations and some are extremely poisonous and can even cause death. If you are picking wild, take an expert with you

HERBS: GROW YOUR OWN

Fresh is best, but dried herbs have their place, too. Here are the 12 disciples to get you started.

DILL

Dark mossy green, this feathery bitter herb is loved by the Scandinavians – what would gravadlax be without its pretty green border? – and Eastern Europeans alike, its grassy sourness balancing creamy potato salads, soups and more. Add to double-podded broad beans, natural yoghurt, olive oil, lemon juice and seasoning.

CHIVES

Chives' tender, hollow blades can be snipped using scissors straight into its chosen destination – a cheesy omelette, a sour cream-loaded jacket potato, or fish chowder. They're pretty useless for cooking so keep them for garnish and make the most of the crowning purple flowers too, which have the same mild allium flavour.

BASIL

A delicate herb, which bruises and blackens easily, so only eat fresh, gently pick the leaves from its stalk and tear or slice with a super-sharp knife, adding to meals right at the last minute or raw.

MINT

It's so easy to grow it's best done in containers – and is a winner in food and drink. Bruise whole stalks of spearmint into Mojitos with rum, or steep peppermint in hot water for tea. Finely chop into Middle Eastern tabbouleh with chunks of salty Feta, or add to braised butter beans and pancetta.

OREGANO

Oregano is one of the few soft herbs that can still be used to great effect when dried. Hang bunches to dehydrate and crumble into rich tomato ragus or sprinkle whole fresh leaves over roasted aubergine slices with nuggets of goat's cheese and toasted pine nuts. If using dried add at the beginning of cooking, fresh at the middle or end.

THYME

Woodier herbs such as thyme, naturally lend themselves to the intensity of being dried, working in everything from pasta to roast chicken, but also in sweet dishes too. The slightly floral note behind thyme is great in cakes, particularly with lemon and almonds, and be sure to look out for the fragrant lemon thyme.

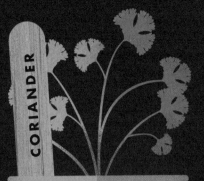

CORIANDER

Some people call it soapy, others zesty and aromatic, but regardless it is thought to be the most widely consumed herb around the world. Its roots are commonly used in Thai green curry pastes; while the fragrant leaves can be sprinkled, sliced or blended into a variety of dishes fresh. A must in guacamole.

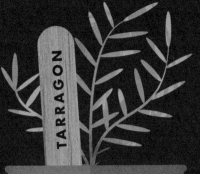

TARRAGON

Best friends with chicken and the secret behind Béarnaise sauce, the soft, shiny narrow leaves of tarragon (particularly the French variety) are intensely aniseed. Like basil and mint, it's a delicate soul, so don't hack at it with a blunt knife once you've picked the leaves from the stalk.

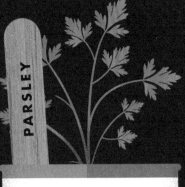

PARSLEY

This umbelliferous leaf is fresh, almost grassy, complements so much and the star of many a show. Try Italy's salsa verde, the raw garnish gremolata, Argentinian chimichurri or England's creamy parsley sauce. Choose flat-leaf above curly.

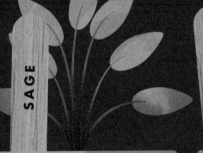

SAGE

Unpleasant to eat on its own thanks to its downy texture and slight bitterness, it's best cooked for long periods of time, say in pork stuffing, or fried in butter until crisp and intensely savoury. It loves meat like veal, pork and bacon, and offal such as liver, but also substantial vegetables such as squash and beets.

ROSEMARY

Robust rosemary gives great fragrance to dishes and should be added early on. Finely chopped leaves are best or add whole, stalks and all, then remove before serving. Infuse stocks, sauces and stews, or use as edible skewers and pierce marinated chicken pieces or paneer before barbecuing.

BAY

The toughest of all the herbs but a great natural aromatic, bay leaves are a store cupboard essential. There's little difference between fresh or dried, but add whole at the beginning of cooking to infuse with its subtle spiciness and remove before serving – it adds a lovely note to creamy puddings as well.

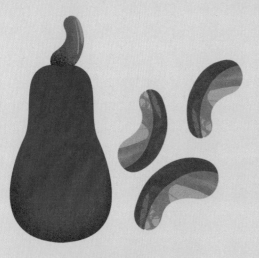

BUTTER

Blended until smooth and spreadable on their own or with a combo of ingredients (think hazelnut and chocolate or peanut and chilli)

CHEESE

Naturally creamy nuts such as Brazil, macadamia and cashews all make great soft and medium-hard 'cheeses' through blending (often with the addition of 'cheesy' nutritional yeast) and sometimes straining

FROM THE PLOT
——

NUTS: TO GO CRAZY FOR

There's so much more to nature's snack than the salted peanuts you find in bars around the world. Raw, they are a pure source of energy, rich in heart-healthy fats, muscle-building and -repairing protein and skin-loving vitamin E. Each has its own nutritional make-up, flavour, texture and appearance but as a collective, nuts are essential in a cook's

CASHEWS

Why are cashews so expensive? Cashew nuts are attached to a cashew apple – a bitter fruit (although the juice is sweet) that has a very short shelf life. The nut part is usually roasted whole and then cracked open to reveal the buttery, sweet kernel inside

MILK/CREAM

Soaked nuts, drained, blended with double the volume of fresh water, and strained – dairy alternative, smoothie essential, delicious in porridge

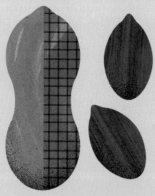

PEANUTS

Peanuts are actually a legume – growing from a plant on the ground like a bean, rather than trees like other nuts

FLOUR

Chestnut flour is rich and sweet, and ideal for gluten-free baking

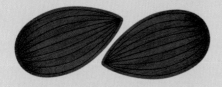

ALMONDS

Almonds are the US's largest speciality crop export and their favourite nut to consume (ranking well above peanuts, walnuts, pecans and pistachios)

GROUND

Great in everything from cakes to curries

CRUNCH TIME

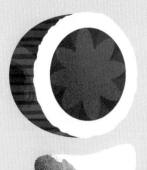

WHOLE, RAW

As nature intended –
the perfect, portable
nutritious snack

BRAZILS

Brazil nuts are encased in an ouriço,
about the size of a coconut, and packed
in like segments of an orange. These
nuts are high in selenium, a mineral
essential to our health, boosting our
immunity and more

larder. From the naturally
creamy macadamia nuts from
Australia, or sweet pecans from North
America, to bitter walnuts and crunchy
peanuts that add significant texture
and flavour to as many savoury
dishes as they do sweet.

Whole nuts last best in airtight
containers at room temperature, so if
you need nibbed or ground buy little
and often, while the starchy chestnut
(which has significantly less oil than
its crunchy counterparts) is best
bought in vacuum packs or
ready puréed if not fresh and
in season.

WHOLE, TOASTED

Toasting in a dry pan or
in the oven until golden,
develops flavour and
crunch

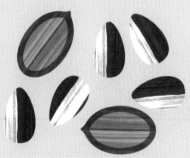

SEEDS

Seeds such as pine nuts, sunflower
seeds and pumpkin seeds are also
great sources of nutrition and can add
another dimension to your cooking.
Toast whole or grind into butters,
pastes and pesto

FLAKED

Flaked almonds and
coconut work well
in baking

CHOPPED/ NIBBED

Salads and sauces,
biscuits and breads –
up the texture
and taste

PISTACHIOS

Chlorophyll makes pistachios the
uniquely green nut – the darker the
green, the better the nut. (Iranian
pistachios are particularly good)

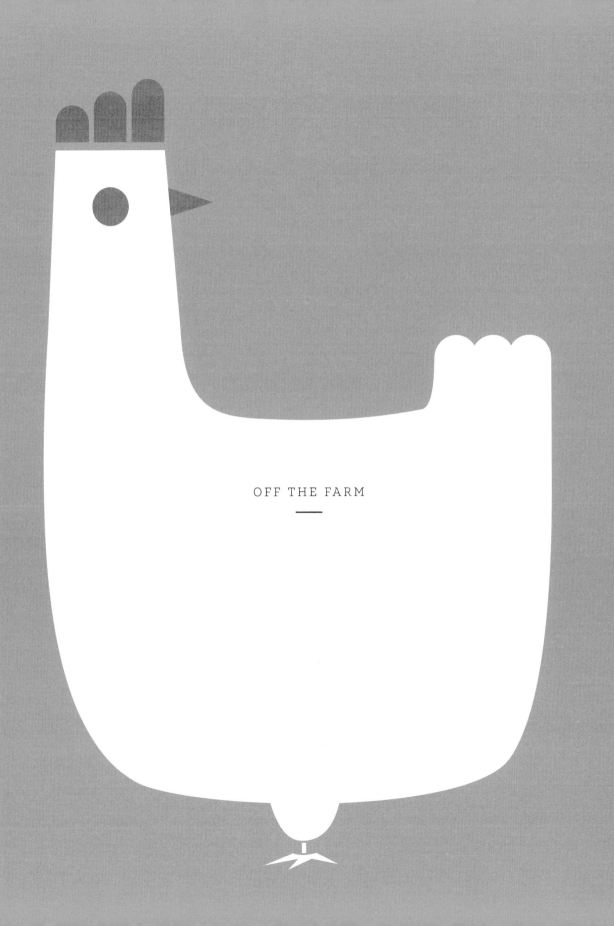

OFF THE FARM
—

Look out for
grass-fed beef
above grain-fed for
superior flavour

For the best results, oil the
steak and not the pan before
frying or grilling and ensure
the pan/grill is smoking hot
before adding the meat

Season beef
well just before
cooking

Beef benefits from
ageing to develop its
flavour and tenderize
the meat. It can be
'dry-aged' or more
commonly 'wet-aged'
for at least 21 days

OFF THE FARM

—

BEEF: WHO'S GOT IT?

Look out for a deep
and even carmine
red colour to the
meat

When we talk about beef the majority of us will be referring to
the meat of castrated male cattle, known as steers and bullocks,
that are slaughtered between one-and-a-half and two years old.
Younger male calves, up to a year old, are sold as veal, while female
dairy cows keep us stocked up in milk, butter, cream and cheese. But,
how do these mighty animals translate as food on our plates?

Marbling of fat
is a good thing
if you like your
meat tender and
full of flavour

Different countries approach breaking down the carcass in their
own way. The French are renowned for seam butchery – following the
natural lines of the animal's muscles – while traditionally Brits and, in a
similar way, Americans, keep things simple – cutting straight, through bone
and fat, to create roasting and grilling joints.

Generally, where the animal has had to work hard (think the front,
forequarter) the meat will be tougher, requiring long and slow-cooking
techniques; such as braising or stewing. The middle of the animal, between
hoof and horn, is where you'll find the good stuff – cuts such as sirloin, fillet
and rump – that can be quickly pan-fried and served as steak.

Don't dismiss the 'other' bits though: bones can be used for stock, while
marrow is delicious roasted and spread on toast with salt. Oxtail and cheek
are exceptionally succulent and flavourful when braised; quickly sautéed
liver is a thing of beauty when perched upon a bed of creamy mash, while
even the testicles are a delicacy known as Rocky Mountain oysters.

Beef should be
brought up to
room temperature
before cooking

Different cuts of steak suit
different levels of cooking
but all should be well rested
in a warm place to allow the
meat to 'relax' and become as
juicy as possible

The fat should
be the colour of
cream, not yellow,
and firm to touch

Caramelisation = flavour. 'Browning' beef,
either as steak, a whole roasting joint or
chunks for a stew, will up your flavour game

TASTY SLICE: KNOW YOUR STEAK

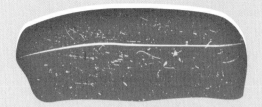

Feather blade

From the shoulder, cheap, best cooked
fast and rare, or slow braised

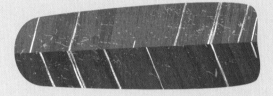

Hanger

From the 'plate' of the cow with an almost
offally flavour, best butterflied before cooking,
cooked medium-rare and sliced thinly

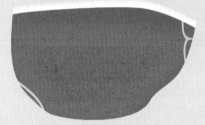

Rump

Backside of the cow, great flavour but
not as tender as fillet, so best cooked
medium-rare or medium

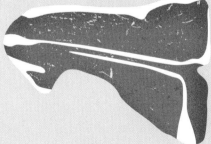

T-bone

Best of both worlds! On the bone:
part fillet, part sirloin; aim to cook
medium-rare

Fillet

From the middle back, lean (and so less
flavourful) but tender, best cooked rare

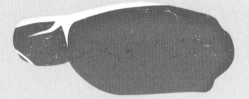

Sirloin

From the middle back, ensure you
cook the border of fat as well as the
meat medium-rare

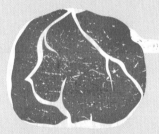

Rib-eye

Found in the fore rib, with great
marbling of fat (i.e. flavour!), best
cooked medium-rare

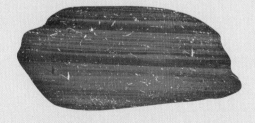

Skirt

From the diaphragm, with well-worked
muscles, cook rare to medium-rare and slice
against the grain for the tenderest cut

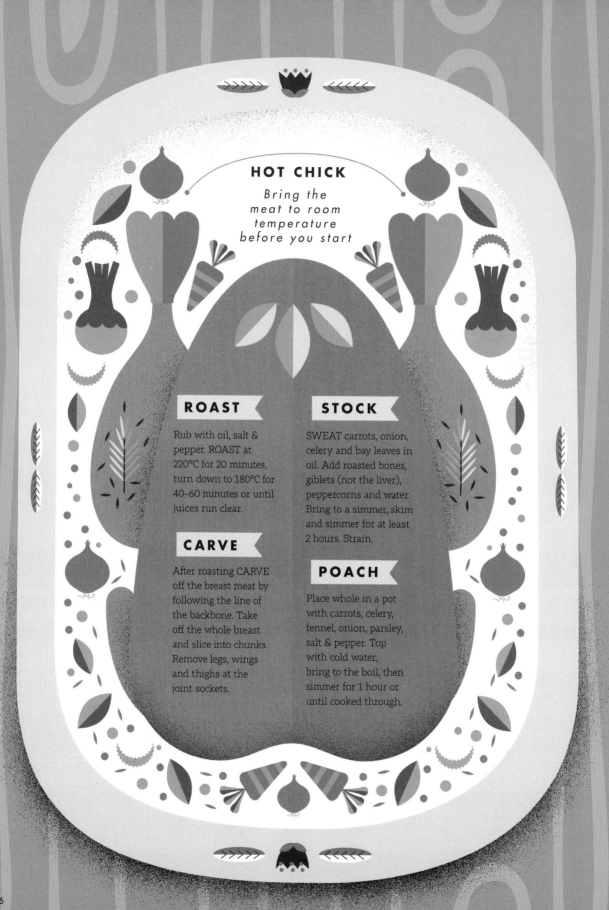

HOT CHICK

Bring the meat to room temperature before you start

ROAST

Rub with oil, salt & pepper. ROAST at 220°C for 20 minutes, turn down to 180°C for 40–60 minutes or until juices run clear.

STOCK

SWEAT carrots, onion, celery and bay leaves in oil. Add roasted bones, giblets (not the liver), peppercorns and water. Bring to a simmer, skim and simmer for at least 2 hours. Strain.

CARVE

After roasting CARVE off the breast meat by following the line of the backbone. Take off the whole breast and slice into chunks. Remove legs, wings and thighs at the joint sockets.

POACH

Place whole in a pot with carrots, celery, fennel, onion, parsley, salt & pepper. Top with cold water, bring to the boil, then simmer for 1 hour or until cooked through.

CHICKEN: FOWL PLAY

As the second most consumed meat in the world (pork takes the top spot), chicken unsurprisingly is the key ingredient to some of our favourite dishes. Its inoffensive, comfortingly bland flavour works grilled, roasted, fried or poached; on its own, or drowned in spice; and is great for those that like to waste little.

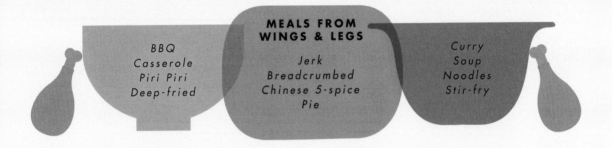

MEALS FROM WINGS & LEGS

BBQ
Casserole
Piri Piri
Deep-fried

Jerk
Breadcrumbed
Chinese 5-spice
Pie

Curry
Soup
Noodles
Stir-fry

WE ARE EATING:

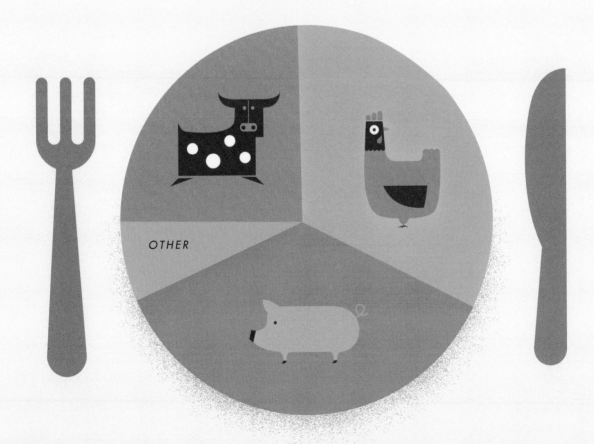

OTHER

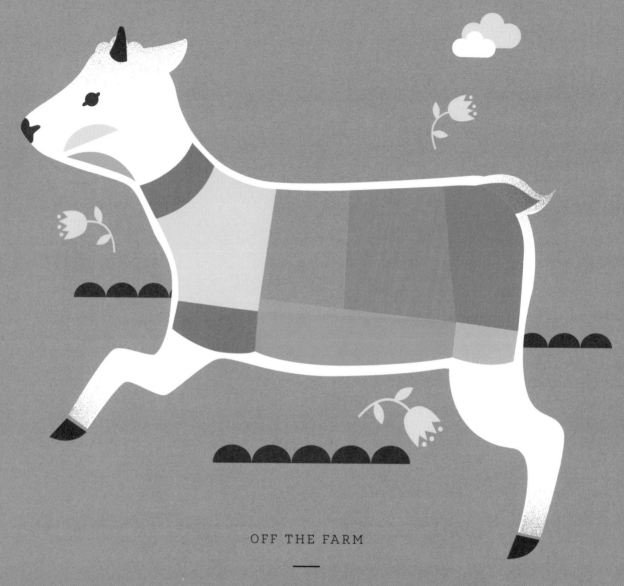

LAMB: SHEEPISH

Whether minced, gently seasoned with cinnamon and layered with aubergine and a rich béchamel in a Greek moussaka or roasted, sliced and blushing, and swimming in mint sauce for a Sunday lunch, lamb is a meat that is as versatile as it is widely loved.

Favoured for its distinctive flavour and sweet fat, lamb is classified as the meat of a sheep under 12 months old, and China, Australia and New Zealand are the biggest producers in the world, closely followed by India and the UK. It's loved in Europe in various guises. The Italians celebrate Easter with abbacchio, a milk-fed lamb barely a month old, its meat tender and pale, similar to veal. In northern Spain they roast their suckling lechazo whole; while the Turkish (and much of the Middle East, actually) like theirs minced and spiced in a kofta kebab.

It's a meat that's strong enough to cope with spice (that's why I'll always opt for a lamb curry on a Friday night) and pairs well with dried fruits (in slow-cooked tagines). Lamb gets even better with flavour the older it is and benefits from hanging after slaughter, like its mate

BUTCHER'S CUTS KEY

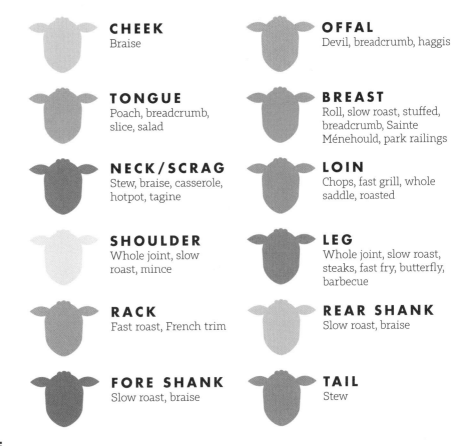

CHEEK
Braise

OFFAL
Devil, breadcrumb, haggis

TONGUE
Poach, breadcrumb, slice, salad

BREAST
Roll, slow roast, stuffed, breadcrumb, Sainte Ménehould, park railings

NECK/SCRAG
Stew, braise, casserole, hotpot, tagine

LOIN
Chops, fast grill, whole saddle, roasted

SHOULDER
Whole joint, slow roast, mince

LEG
Whole joint, slow roast, steaks, fast fry, butterfly, barbecue

RACK
Fast roast, French trim

REAR SHANK
Slow roast, braise

FORE SHANK
Slow roast, braise

TAIL
Stew

A SHEEP'S LIFE

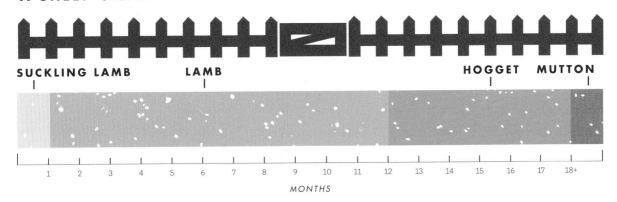

SUCKLING LAMB LAMB HOGGET MUTTON

1 2 3 4 5 6 7 8 9 10 11 12 13 14 15 16 17 18+

MONTHS

beef. It also takes on the flavour of its natural environment. Grass-fed lamb is always preferable over grain, but if you can try salt-marsh lamb from the UK that dines on a combination of samphire, sorrel and sea lavender, or saltbush lamb from Oz, with its penchant for old man saltbush, do.

In some countries, you'll find hogget (when the sheep is slaughtered around 12–18 months)

but it's mutton that gets really interesting. After 18 months the meat darkens and strengthens in flavour. Yes, it might get tougher, but that allows for long and slow cooking. Britain's Prince Charles loves the stuff – so much so, in fact, that he's been campaigning for a 'mutton renaissance' since 2004. Indeed, it's a traditional ingredient for many of our favourite dishes today – even if

cheaper-to-produce lamb has now taken its place – such as North Africa's rich, spiced merguez sausage, Irish stew, Welsh cawl, Icelandic smoked and boiled hangikjöt (traditionally served with béchamel at Christmas) and English hotpot from Lancashire, which originally was joined by kidneys and oysters underneath its famous buttery sliced potato topping.

SAUSAGE: THE BIG BANGER THEORY

The world of sausages is a colourful and characterful one. They can come fresh or dried, smoked or cooked; meaty, fishy or veggie; packed with herbs and spices, or even bulging with blood. Whichever way they come, they've found a home on our little planet. While most sausages began life as a way of preserving our hunt, from Scottish haggis to Italian salami, we're talking about fresh sausages here. They're the ones you barbeque in the summer, grill of a Saturday morning for a classic English fry-up, or roast in the oven with a Yorkshire pudding batter for a traditional 'toad-in-the-hole'. These sausages usually consist of minced meat (most often pork, but beef, lamb and poultry can also make an appearance), fat (particularly in Britain where the ideal meat to fat ratio is around 75:25), spices and herbs (specific to a region), salt (to season and help preserve) and casing (naturally the animal's intestines, but modern mass-produced sausages sometimes use artificial 'skins'). Often the scraps and leftovers of the animal, after the prime cuts have been taken, are used to make sausages. But as one of Britain's great butchers once told me (Marc-Frederic, aka the Sausage Doctor), there are no mistakes in butchery, just more sausages.

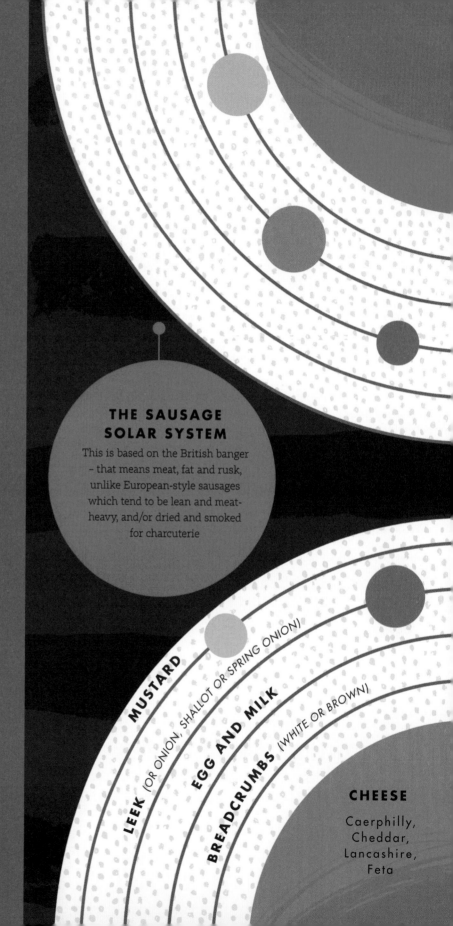

THE SAUSAGE SOLAR SYSTEM

This is based on the British banger – that means meat, fat and rusk, unlike European-style sausages which tend to be lean and meat-heavy, and/or dried and smoked for charcuterie

MUSTARD

LEEK (OR ONION, SHALLOT OR SPRING ONION)

EGG AND MILK

BREADCRUMBS (WHITE OR BROWN)

CHEESE

Caerphilly, Cheddar, Lancashire, Feta

MEAT
Pork, beef, lamb, veal, offal

FAT

RUSK (OR BREADCRUMBS)

SPICES AND HERBS

SALT

CASING

PLANET VEGGIE
Don't fancy meat? Try a take on the Welsh recipe for Glamorgan sausages, which celebrate leek and cheese in all their gastronomic glory

THE BIG BANG
To prick or not to prick your sausage, that's the question. I say nay. Sausages with natural casings shouldn't split. The trick is to pan-fry them low and slow until golden all over and cooked

CHARCUTERIE: HOW'S IT HANGING?

Just as squirrels (aptly) squirrel away nuts to see them through the winter, throughout history us humans have looked to preserve our hunts.

Through the addition of salt and/ or smoke to meat (as well as fish and vegetables), we discovered that we could make our food last longer and taste rather good too. Indeed, so superior was this cured flavour that even with the modern refrigeration and freezing techniques that we have today, we still practice these traditional methods.

Charcuterie, as we now know it, first boomed in 15th-century France. While the methods might have been used since the ancient civilizations, it was here that guilds of pork butchers, or 'charcutiers', developed many of the recipes that we eat now – from saucisson and jambon to pâté.

Of course, curing meat is as much about good butchery as clever chemistry. Sodium chloride (salt), is crucial to the preserving process. It's all about keeping the bad bacteria out and good bacteria in (through osmosis and dehydration), enhancing and intensifying flavour (through controlled fermentation) and tenderization (by breaking down of the proteins). Most meats need 2% to 5% salt for this process (anything over will taste 'salty'). You can also add hot or cold smoke, sugar (which are both antibacterial), spice and fat; crucial for flavour and texture.

TAKE ONE

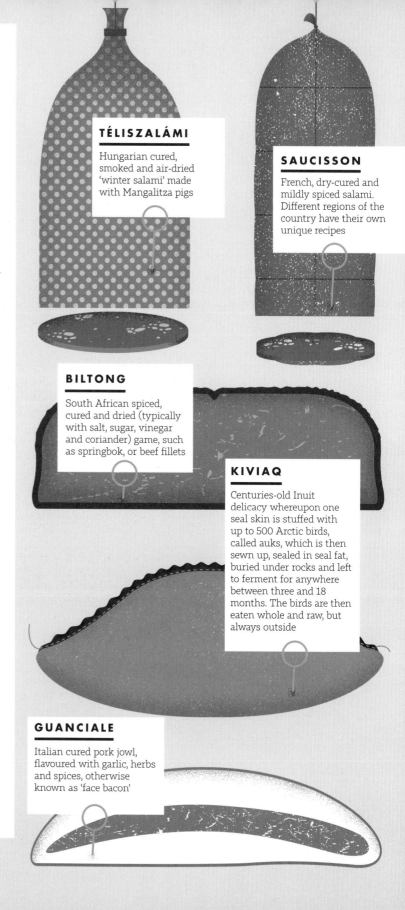

TÉLISZALÁMI

Hungarian cured, smoked and air-dried 'winter salami' made with Mangalitza pigs

SAUCISSON

French, dry-cured and mildly spiced salami. Different regions of the country have their own unique recipes

BILTONG

South African spiced, cured and dried (typically with salt, sugar, vinegar and coriander) game, such as springbok, or beef fillets

KIVIAQ

Centuries-old Inuit delicacy whereupon one seal skin is stuffed with up to 500 Arctic birds, called auks, which is then sewn up, sealed in seal fat, buried under rocks and left to ferment for anywhere between three and 18 months. The birds are then eaten whole and raw, but always outside

GUANCIALE

Italian cured pork jowl, flavoured with garlic, herbs and spices, otherwise known as 'face bacon'

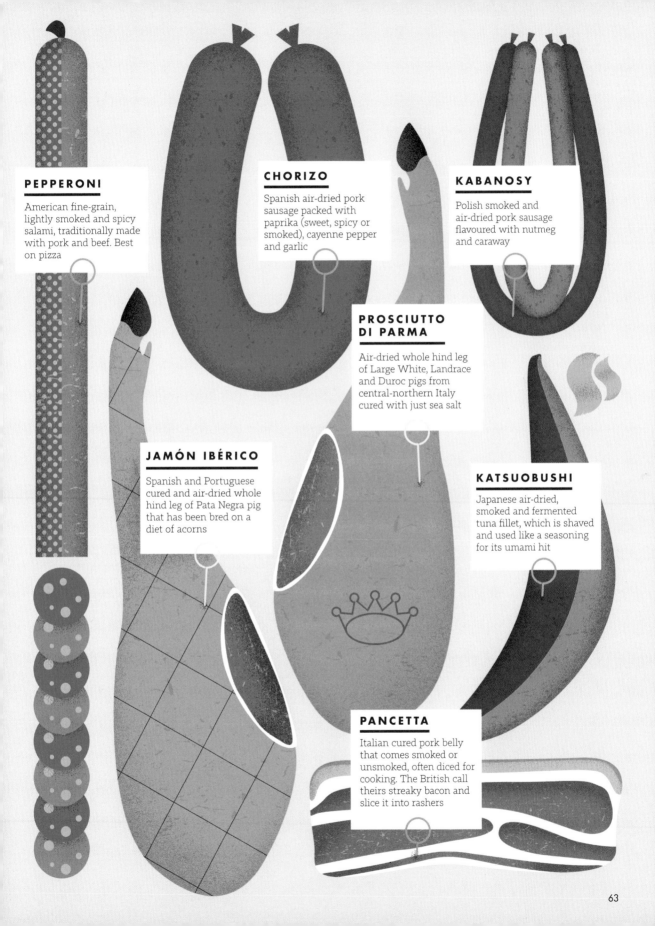

PEPPERONI

American fine-grain, lightly smoked and spicy salami, traditionally made with pork and beef. Best on pizza

CHORIZO

Spanish air-dried pork sausage packed with paprika (sweet, spicy or smoked), cayenne pepper and garlic

KABANOSY

Polish smoked and air-dried pork sausage flavoured with nutmeg and caraway

PROSCIUTTO DI PARMA

Air-dried whole hind leg of Large White, Landrace and Duroc pigs from central-northern Italy cured with just sea salt

JAMÓN IBÉRICO

Spanish and Portuguese cured and air-dried whole hind leg of Pata Negra pig that has been bred on a diet of acorns

KATSUOBUSHI

Japanese air-dried, smoked and fermented tuna fillet, which is shaved and used like a seasoning for its umami hit

PANCETTA

Italian cured pork belly that comes smoked or unsmoked, often diced for cooking. The British call their streaky bacon and slice it into rashers

BLOOD: THE MOST UNDERVALUED INGREDIENT

Not all ingredients are made equal but blood, so often seen as a by-product of the meat industry, is certainly one undervalued. A rich source of protein and iron, it is the foundation of sausages around the world – from Britain's spicy breakfast favourite 'black pudding' and Spain's soft 'morcilla' to Estonia's Christmas banger 'verivorstid'. It's strong metallic flavour means it stands up well to punchy spices and herbs.

The Maasai tribe of Tanzania likes to drink blood straight from the cow's neck, mixed with milk, while Inuits prefer downing seal blood. Asia tends to use duck or pig's blood traditionally; whether set and sliced like tofu in China; combined with rice, steamed and seasoned into savoury cakes as street food in Taiwan, or chilled and coagulated in a raw soup as in North Vietnam.

In Europe, the Polish combine duck blood with the meat of the bird, spices, dried fruits and vinegar for a warming czarnina, while Italians mix theirs into a sweet chocolate pudding flavoured with orange and cinnamon, called sanguinaccio. It's also a natural thickener for sauces and stews – old-school French add it to coq au vin.

The Finnish choose to eat their blood sausage with lingonberry sauce and are famous for their blood pancakes, which are served across much of Scandinavia. Indeed, research in 2014 by the Nordic Food Lab showed that many dishes featuring eggs could actually use animal blood as a replacement. Both feature albumin proteins and so react in a similar way when exposed to heat or with the introduction of air through whipping – we're talking meringues, macarons, pasta, custard, ice cream and even cakes, all taking on a suspiciously darker hue…

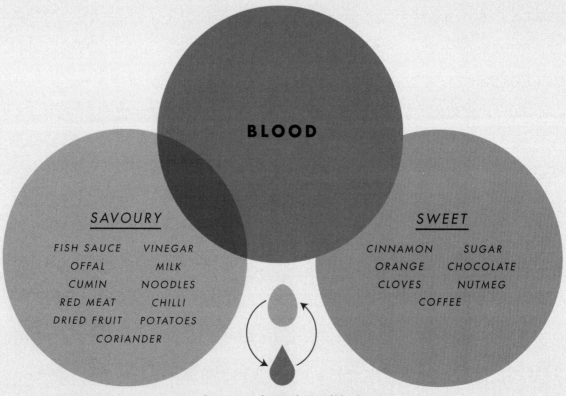

BLOOD

SAVOURY

FISH SAUCE   VINEGAR
OFFAL   MILK
CUMIN   NOODLES
RED MEAT   CHILLI
DRIED FRUIT   POTATOES
CORIANDER

SWEET

CINNAMON   SUGAR
ORANGE   CHOCOLATE
CLOVES   NUTMEG
COFFEE

Swap 1 egg white with 43g of blood

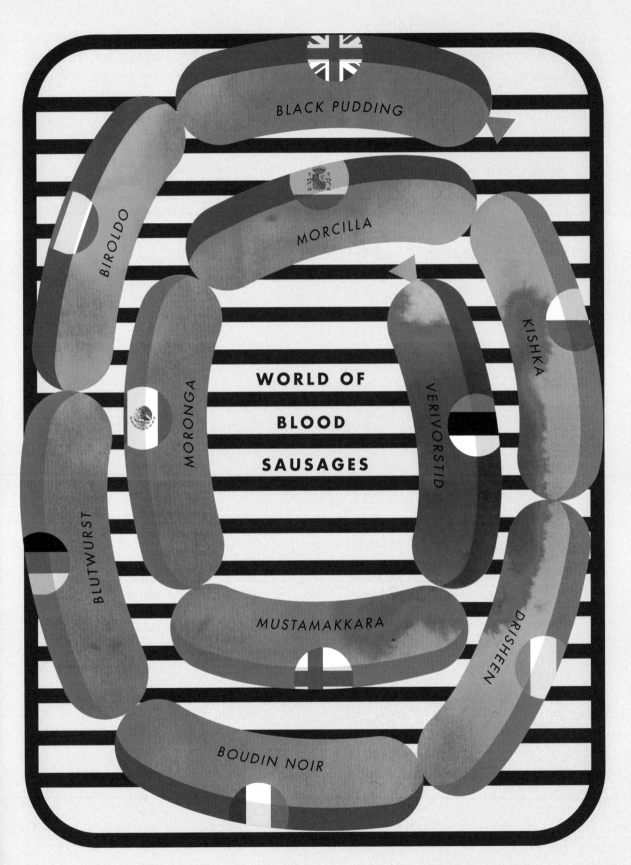

WORLD OF BLOOD SAUSAGES

BLACK PUDDING

MORCILLA

BIROLDO

KISHKA

MORONGA

VERIVORSTID

BLUTWURST

MUSTAMAKKARA

DRISHEEN

BOUDIN NOIR

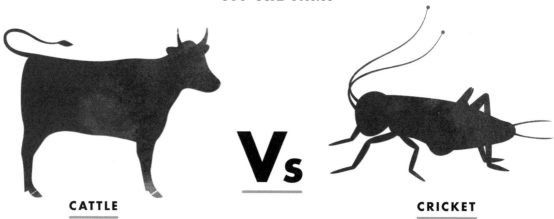

CATTLE Vs **CRICKET**

Crickets need 12 x less feed than cattle

80% of a cricket is edible vs 40% of a cow

Crickets contain 8–25g/100g protein vs 19-26g/100g in raw beef

Crickets need less water, less feed, less land and less pesticides than cattle

INSECTS: TRY BEFORE YOU DIE

In Western cultures creepy crawlies are just that – scary little beasties that fly, jump, bite and live in the most unappealing places. They're certainly not the pre-cut steaks, cellophaned and presented on the supermarket shelf that we're used to. But eating bugs really is nothing new.

As a report by the Food and Agriculture Organization in 2013 proved, 28% of the globe's population is already nibbling at all manner of beetles, bees, grasshoppers, caterpillars, dragonflies and more, at various stages in their life cycles. Some are 'famine foods', eaten during lean times or rainy seasons for their high protein, iron and zinc content, but many are enjoyed as delicacies for their varied tastes and textures. Aboriginal Australians are renowned for their love of creamy witchetty grubs, which can be eaten raw or cooked; while in Thailand it is crunchy red ants, and their eggs, which find themselves in various salads and omelettes.

They make environmental sense too, as well as being surprisingly nutritious. While most are currently harvested from the wild, farmed insects emit considerably fewer greenhouse gases than traditional livestock, they can be fed on organic waste and take up much less space.

After all, who thought it was a good idea to first eat lobster; are locusts not just land shrimps by another name?

Species of edible insects.........................1900

People already eating insects as part of their traditional diet..........2 billion

Amount of insects to every human.........40 tonnes

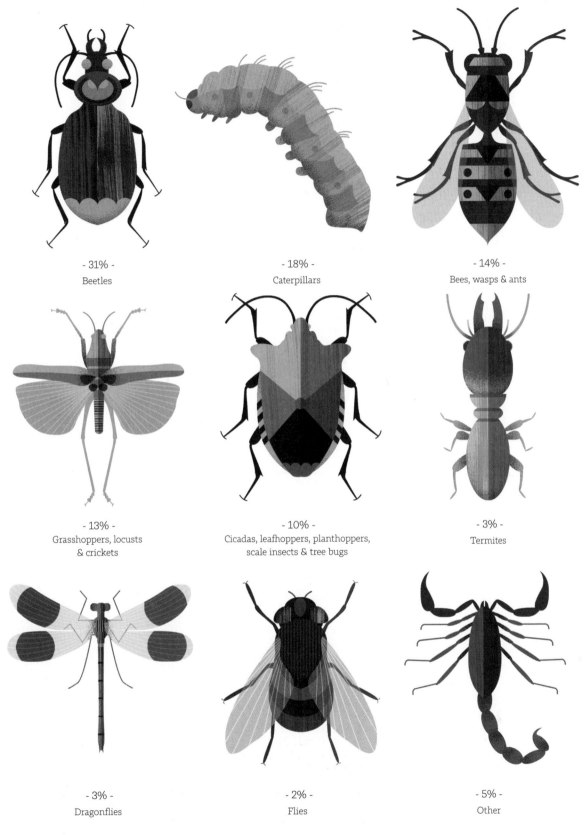

- 31% -
Beetles

- 18% -
Caterpillars

- 14% -
Bees, wasps & ants

- 13% -
Grasshoppers, locusts
& crickets

- 10% -
Cicadas, leafhoppers, planthoppers,
scale insects & tree bugs

- 3% -
Termites

- 3% -
Dragonflies

- 2% -
Flies

- 5% -
Other

% APPROXIMATE INSECTS EATEN GLOBALLY

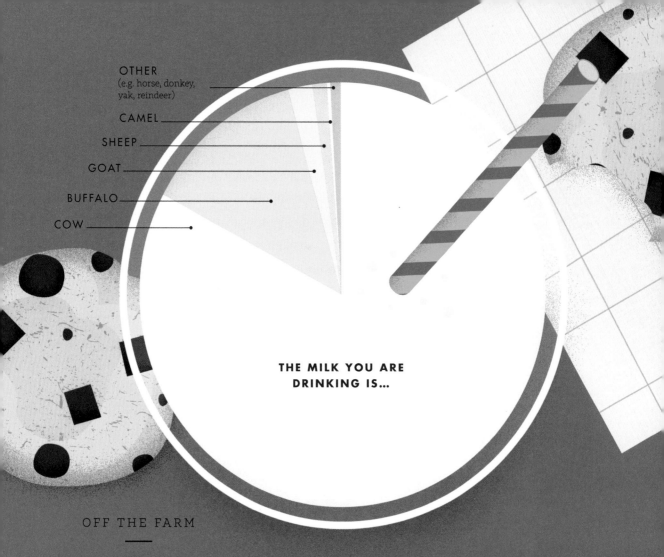

OTHER
(e.g. horse, donkey,
yak, reindeer)

CAMEL

SHEEP

GOAT

BUFFALO

COW

**THE MILK YOU ARE
DRINKING IS...**

OFF THE FARM

___

MILK: THE
WHITE STUFF

More than six billion of us around the world enjoy the white stuff, whether in its purest form, as milk, or transformed into cream, butter, cheese or yoghurt. Dairy is big business.

The majority of milk we drink is derived from cattle but other animals can be successfully milked too – from the more familiar sheep and goat, to (perhaps surprisingly) horses and even camels. And while

the nutritious content of each varies, fresh milk is undeniably a worthwhile addition to our diet. Cow's milk, in particular, is a great source of protein, calcium and a whole host of vitamins.

The average dairy cow can produce enough milk in a day to fill up a car tank

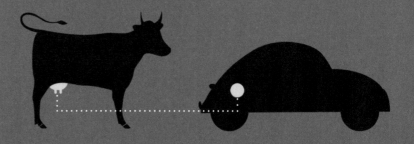

NUTS
SEEDS
(almonds,
coconuts,
sunflower
seeds etc.)

OATS

SOY

RICE

WHAT DOES IT MEAN?

RAW

Completely untreated and unheated milk – i.e. straight from the udder! The distribution of raw milk is banned and restricted in some countries due to the potential health risks.

HOMOGENIZATION

Where milk is forced at high pressure through small holes to break up its natural fat globules to ensure an even liquid and no separate cream layer.

PASTEURIZED

Pasteurized is the most common treatment and sees the milk heated to a high temperature and then quickly cooled and bottled to kill potential bacteria and help extend shelf life. The flavour and nutrition of the milk aren't greatly affected.

UHT

UHT stands for ultra-heat-treated milk, and is heated to around double the temperature of pasteurized milk for extra-long shelf life. Flavour and nutrition are affected.

EVAPORATED

Where milk is heated, sterilized and concentrated to half that of standard milk. Thick in texture, and cooked in flavour.

CONDENSED

Much like evaporated milk but sugar is added. A sticky, sweet, thick affair and the basis of delicious dulce de leche and quick fudge.

No.
ONE

India is the world's largest producer of milk

50%
MORE

World milk production increased by more than 50% in the last 30 years

BUTTER: WHIP IT GOOD

To me there are two types of people in the world – butter people (they like to have fun) and margarine people (let's just call them less fun). Having always pitched happily in the former camp, I discovered a world where butter was far more than just a spread for toast or a filler for a baked potato. It was a transformer of vegetables, the starter (and finisher, for that matter) of sauces, the fluffiness of cakes and the flavour behind a truly good omelette.

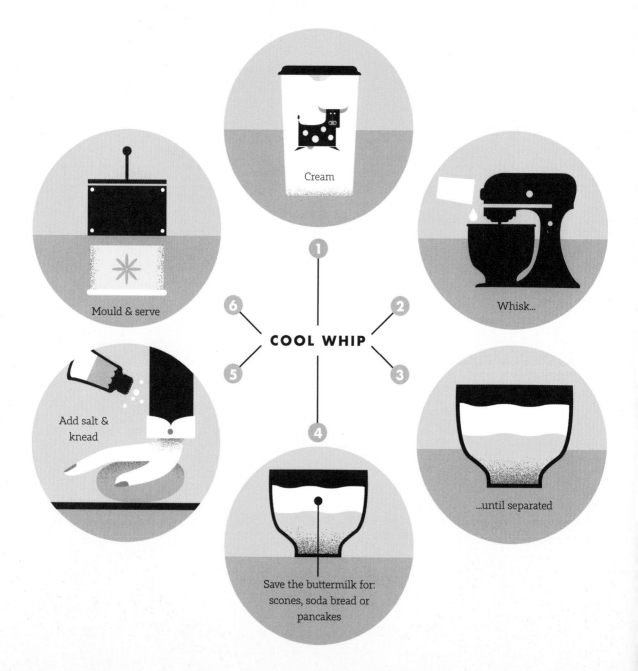

Cream

Whisk...

...until separated

Save the buttermilk for: scones, soda bread or pancakes

Add salt & knead

Mould & serve

COOL WHIP

1
2
3
4
5
6

FLAVOUR SAVER

Infused butters are a great way to inject some added seasoning. The butter must be so soft you can leave a greasy fingerprint, beat it until smooth, then combine with your chosen ingredients. Roll into a sausage shape in greaseproof paper, sealing each end, and refrigerate or freeze. Here are some classics to get you started:

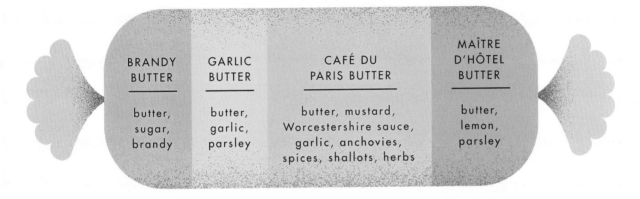

BRANDY BUTTER

butter, sugar, brandy

GARLIC BUTTER

butter, garlic, parsley

CAFÉ DU PARIS BUTTER

butter, mustard, Worcestershire sauce, garlic, anchovies, spices, shallots, herbs

MAÎTRE D'HÔTEL BUTTER

butter, lemon, parsley

BUTTER ME UP

Beurre monté

Beurre blanc

Beurre noir

Beurre noisette

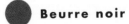 **Beurre monté**

Emulsified butter, made by gradually whisking in cold cubes of butter into simmered water, ideal for poaching meat, fish/shellfish or vegetables, and as a base for other sauces

Beurre blanc

Vinegar, white wine and shallots are reduced, before cold cubes of butter are gradually whisked in to create a hot, pale emulsified butter sauce

Beurre noisette

Butter is melted and allowed to colour until it turns a nut-brown colour. Can be seasoned with lemon, herbs and/or capers, if serving with fish

Beurre noir

Melted butter, as above, that is taken to a dark brown, almost black colour off the heat, again often seasoned with an acid, and famously served with skate

CHEESE: GOING ALL THE WHEY

It's thought that the first cheese was made by happy accident, as milk was transported in the stomachs of animals and the naturally occurring enzymes (called rennet) caused it to separate into solid curds and liquid whey. Either way, it's a process that's barely changed over the thousands of years that we've enjoyed it. Whether fresh, soft and surface-ripened or hard-pressed, cheese is essentially just preserved milk.

Our favourite cheeses are made with cow's milk, and you'll commonly find goat, sheep and even buffalo varieties, but in truth any milk can be made into cheese – from camel and donkey (called pule, the world's most expensive cheese) to human breast milk and (at the opposite end of the scale) almonds and cashews for vegans. It can be smoked, rolled in herbs or aged for years; and once ready can be eaten fresh, sliced into sandwiches, grated into sauces, baked into biscuits or grilled into crispy, blistered deliciousness.

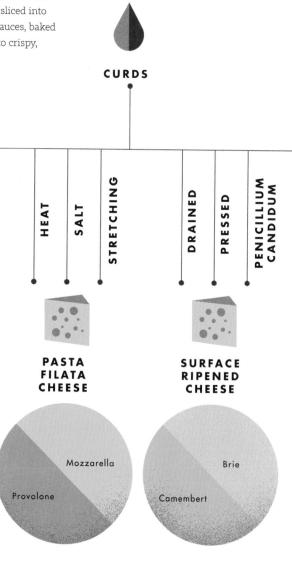

MILK

RENNET

CURDS

DRAINED   PRESSED

DRAINED   PRESSED   BRINED

HEAT   SALT   STRETCHING

DRAINED   PRESSED   PENICILLIUM CANDIDUM

FRESH CHEESE

Cottage Cheese · Quark · Paneer · Cream Cheese · Curd Cheese · Mascarpone

FETA

PASTA FILATA CHEESE

Mozzarella · Provolone

SURFACE RIPENED CHEESE

Brie · Camembert

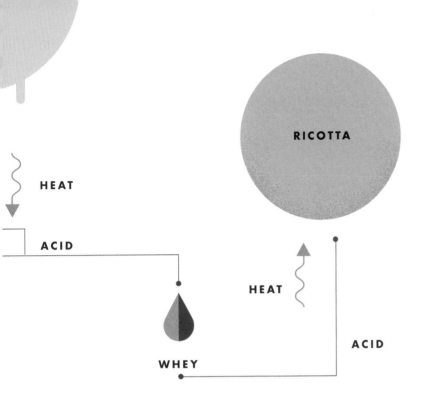

RICOTTA

HEAT

ACID

HEAT

WHEY

ACID

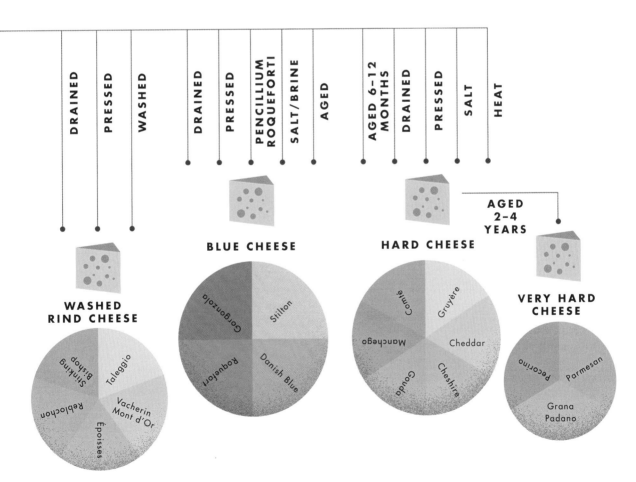

DRAINED

PRESSED

WASHED

DRAINED

PRESSED

PENCILLIUM ROQUEFORTI

SALT/BRINE

AGED

AGED 6–12 MONTHS

DRAINED

PRESSED

SALT

HEAT

AGED 2–4 YEARS

BLUE CHEESE

HARD CHEESE

VERY HARD CHEESE

WASHED RIND CHEESE

Stinking Bishop

Taleggio

Reblochon

Vacherin Mont d'Or

Époisses

Gorgonzola

Stilton

Roquefort

Danish Blue

Comte

Gruyère

Manchego

Cheddar

Gouda

Cheshire

Pecorino

Parmesan

Grana Padano

73

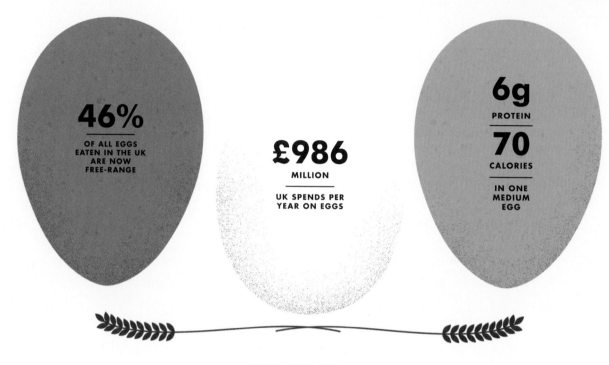

46%
OF ALL EGGS
EATEN IN THE UK
ARE NOW
FREE-RANGE

£986
MILLION

UK SPENDS PER
YEAR ON EGGS

6g
PROTEIN

70
CALORIES

IN ONE
MEDIUM
EGG

—

EGGS: SOURCE TO SAUCE

The humble hen's egg is one of the most readily available, cheap and endlessly versatile food stuffs around, but did you know that it is also one of the most ancient. Us humans have been eating all things ovoid since the Neolithic period, chomping our way through various varieties of fowl egg from chickens, ducks, geese, quail, pheasant, plovers and guinea fowl, to ostriches, emu, pelican, pigeon and gull (the latter is without a fishy taste, despite what some food writers may argue).

It's little wonder, really. The egg is nature's perfectly packaged hand-held, bite-size snack. It's packed with vitamins (A, B, D and E), minerals (iodine, phosphorus, selenium, zinc and iron) and it's a 'complete' protein, meaning that it has all of the essential amino acids that our bodies need. There's a reason Rocky Balboa starts his day by drinking raw eggs...

They are also a cook's friend – delicious in sweet or savoury dishes, whole or separated, on their own or as a component ingredient to bind, set, leaven, thicken, enrich, emulsify, glaze or clarify. They can be boiled (older eggs are best here, as they are easier to peel);

scrambled with butter (slow and low); poached (whisk the water to create a vortex before you crack in a fresh egg); or fried (butter and oil are good, but bacon fat is better). They can also be baked, or shirred as the Americans call it, with cream and topped with cheese and breadcrumbs. And, if you celebrate Jewish Passover, you might even like to roast your egg (Beitzah) until the shell browns and cracks – just make sure you boil it first.

Whatever you do to them, they are best approached at room temperature, particularly in baking. You can check just how fresh they are, too, by placing them carefully in a glass of water. If they sink to the bottom they are good to go, while a floater can be discarded, that is unless you're in China. Thousand-year-eggs are a delicacy here. Preserved in a combination of salt, lime and ashes, the egg is left for 45–100 days, whereupon the white turns yellow, firm and gelatinous, and the yolk, green and cheese-like. It's eaten raw, presumably with noses pinched thanks to the strong smell of ammonia. That's far from the most unusual way to eat eggs, though. Head to South East Asia, specifically the Philippines or Vietnam, and you might stumble across balut – a boiled, fertilized 17–20-day-old duck egg.

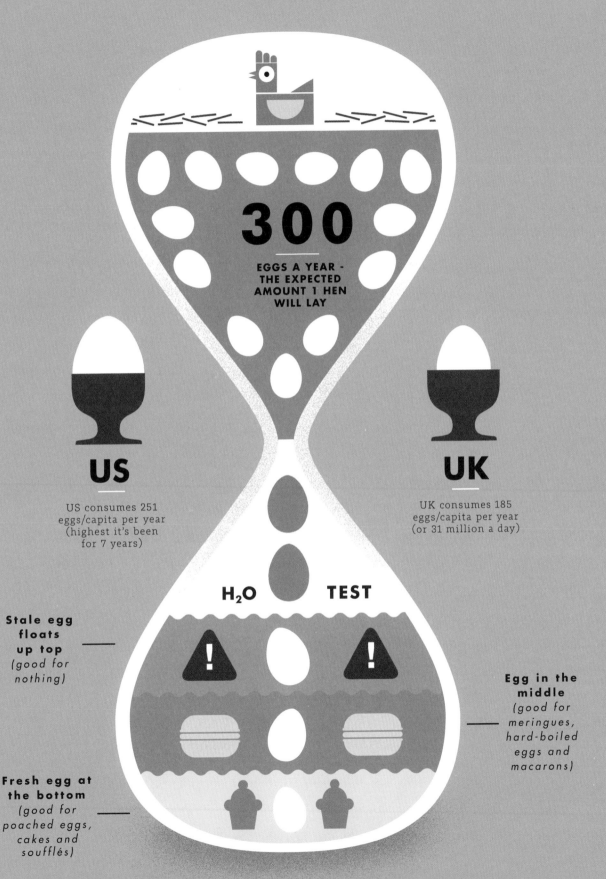

300

EGGS A YEAR -
THE EXPECTED
AMOUNT 1 HEN
WILL LAY

US

US consumes 251
eggs/capita per year
(highest it's been
for 7 years)

UK

UK consumes 185
eggs/capita per year
(or 31 million a day)

H₂O   TEST

**Stale egg
floats
up top**
(good for
nothing)

**Egg in the
middle**
(good for
meringues,
hard-boiled
eggs and
macarons)

**Fresh egg at
the bottom**
(good for
poached eggs,
cakes and
soufflés)

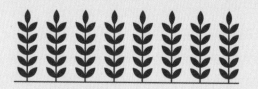

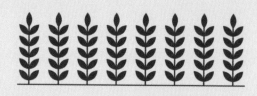

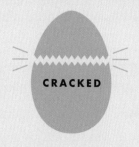
CRACKED

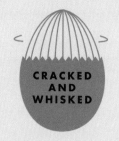
CRACKED AND WHISKED

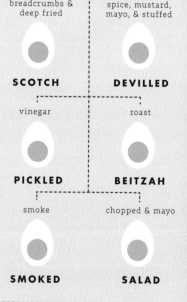
BOILED

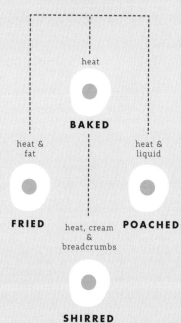

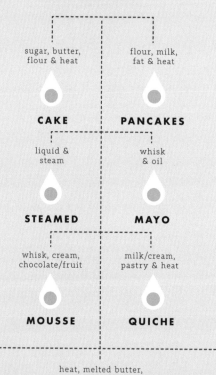

heat
BAKED

sugar, butter, flour & heat
CAKE

flour, milk, fat & heat
PANCAKES

sausagemeat, breadcrumbs & deep fried
SCOTCH

yolk mashed, spice, mustard, mayo, & stuffed
DEVILLED

heat & fat
FRIED

heat & liquid
POACHED

liquid & steam
STEAMED

whisk & oil
MAYO

vinegar
PICKLED

roast
BEITZAH

heat, cream & breadcrumbs
SHIRRED

whisk, cream, chocolate/fruit
MOUSSE

milk/cream, pastry & heat
QUICHE

smoke
SMOKED

chopped & mayo
SALAD

low heat, fat & ingredients
FRITTATA

low heat, fat, onions & potatoes
TORTILLA

heat, melted butter, water & flour
CHOUX PASTRY

heat, butter, sugar & lemon/lime/orange
CURD

high heat & fat
OMELETTE

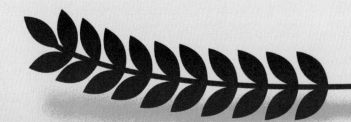

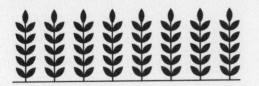

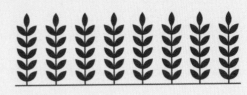

WHITES

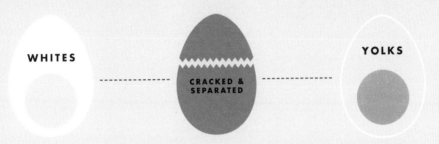

CRACKED & SEPARATED

YOLKS

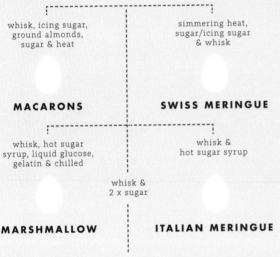

whisk, icing sugar, ground almonds, sugar & heat

simmering heat, sugar/icing sugar & whisk

MACARONS

SWISS MERINGUE

whisk, hot sugar syrup, liquid glucose, gelatin & chilled

whisk & hot sugar syrup

whisk & 2 x sugar

MARSHMALLOW

ITALIAN MERINGUE

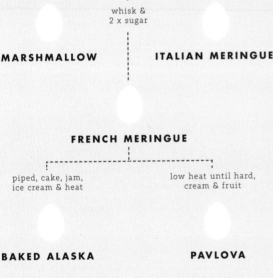

FRENCH MERINGUE

piped, cake, jam, ice cream & heat

low heat until hard, cream & fruit

BAKED ALASKA

PAVLOVA

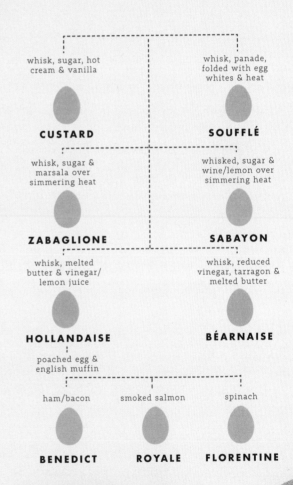

whisk, sugar, hot cream & vanilla

whisk, panade, folded with egg whites & heat

CUSTARD

SOUFFLÉ

whisk, sugar & marsala over simmering heat

whisked, sugar & wine/lemon over simmering heat

ZABAGLIONE

SABAYON

whisk, melted butter & vinegar/ lemon juice

whisk, reduced vinegar, tarragon & melted butter

HOLLANDAISE

BÉARNAISE

poached egg & english muffin

ham/bacon

smoked salmon

spinach

BENEDICT

ROYALE

FLORENTINE

—

HONEY: WHAT'S THE BUZZ ALL ABOUT?

Honey starts life as nectar, which is collected by the honey bee from plants. As the bee swallows the nectar it is converted into simple sugars and it is then delivered to the hive's honeycomb cells. It is here that it evaporates into honey

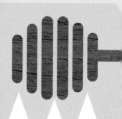

Generally, the lighter the honey in colour, the milder the taste

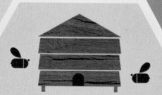

Honey is made by a colony of honey bees – one breeding queen, thousands of male drones (whose sole purpose is to fertilize the queen) and tens of thousands of female worker bees (who do everything else)

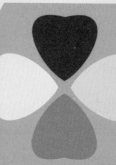

Most mass-produced honey is from bees that have been dining on clover nectar

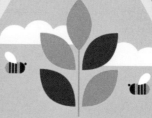

It is thought that around a third of what we eat originates from crops pollinated by insects (80% of which would be bees)

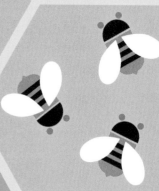

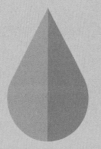

Honey is 18% water

Honey tastes of its environment, whether that be wild herbs or a local avocado crop. Look out for these popular types of honey from around the world, each of which have their own unique colour, flavour and aroma: acacia, eucalyptus, heather, manuka and orange blossom

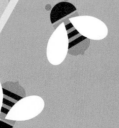

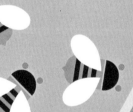

Honey can be used to make mead, beer and liqueurs

20-26°C

Store honey at room temperature to prevent it from crystallizing. If this does occur, submerge a sealed jar of the sweet stuff in hot water and the gentle heat will return it to a pourable liquid

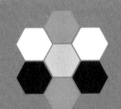

'Raw honey' is honey that hasn't been heated, purified or filtered (to make it clear and liquid) unlike most commercially available honey

Make measuring honey less messy by dipping your spoon in flavourless oil first

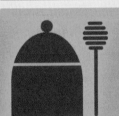

1 bee will produce as little as ¹⁄₁₂ tsp of honey in its lifetime

Honey bees can produce 2-3 times more honey than they need, so it's actually okay for us humans to steal some, as long as we're not too greedy

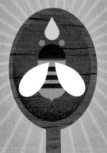

2 million flowers have to be visited by honey bees to make 450g honey (little over 1 jar)

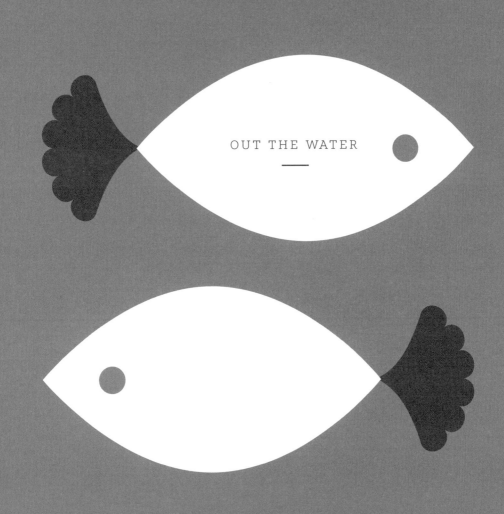

OUT THE WATER

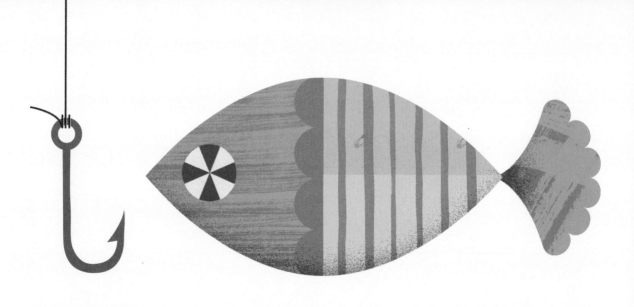

FISH FILLET: SKIN AND SLICE

Unless you catch your own, most of us are used to pre-filleted, pre-portioned, perhaps even golden geometric fingers of our favourite fish. But buying whole is not only often cheaper but you're also more likely to get it fresh and waste less, too. Once you've scaled and gutted your fish, it can be baked or barbecued whole, or you can take the scraps and carcass after filleting and make a stock base for soups and sauces. (Just discard the guts as these can make the stock bitter.)

Most fish can be filleted as shown but if you're unsure ask your fishmonger. Look out for bright eyes, shiny skin, vibrant gills and a fresh ocean smell when buying fish whole. Once it smells 'fishy' it's only good for the cat.

You will need:

A sharp, thin and flexible filleting knife

A pair of fish bone tweezers

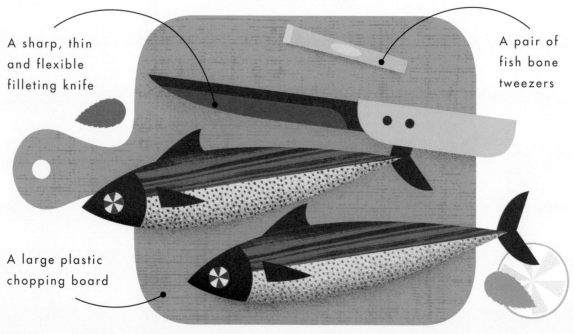

A large plastic chopping board

FILLETING A ROUND FISH

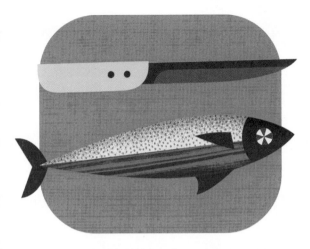

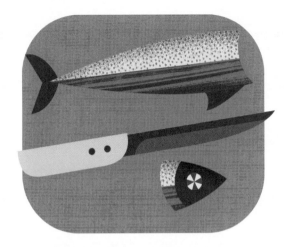

1 Place the fish flat on its side, with the backbone facing you

2 Chop off the head, around the fins

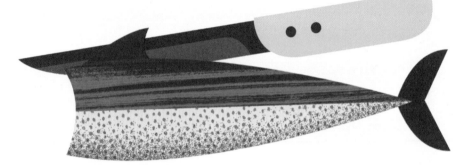

3 Slice along the backbone, using long sweeping cuts, don't saw or hack, until you reach the tail. Keep the knife as close to the bones as possible, let them be your guide, until the fillet comes away

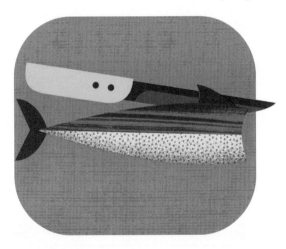

4 Turn the fish over and repeat

5 Some fish may need pin-boning – use tweezers – and trim the two fillets of any unwanted fat or skin

FILLETING A FLAT FISH

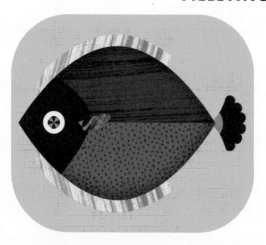

1 Place the fish flat on its belly

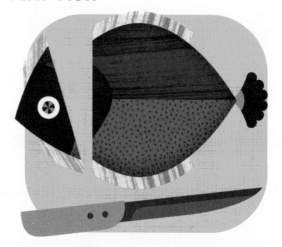

2 Chop off the head

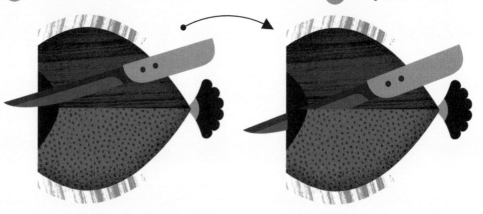

3 Slice along the backbone down to the tail, angle the knife and slice along the bones, using long sweeping cuts, to release the first fillet. Repeat with the adjacent fillet

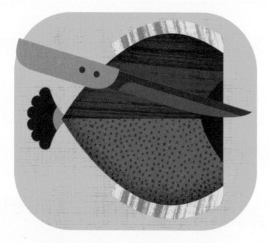

4 Turn the fish over and repeat with the two underside fillets

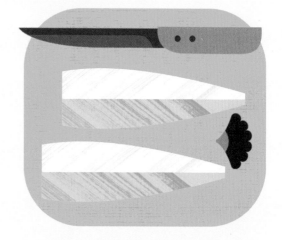

5 Pin-bone, then trim the four fillets of any unwanted fat, fins or skin

SKINNING A FILLET

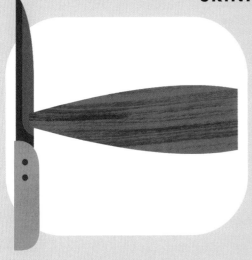
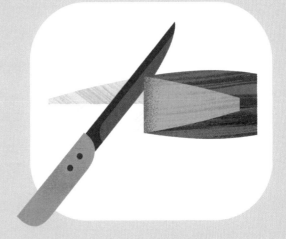

1 Flat or round, skin-side down, take the tail end of the fillet and make a small incision, being careful not to cut through the skin

2 Angle the knife and carefully slice, in a sawing motion, between the fillet and skin. Use the skin as a lever, pulling it taut with every slice until the fillet comes clean away

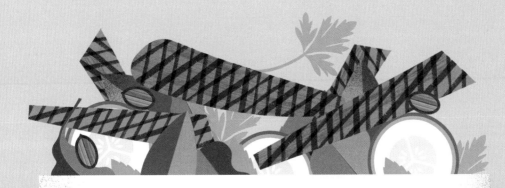

DON'T BIN THE SKIN!

Salmon skin is delicious roasted with salt until crispy like pork crackling. Break into shards to garnish a warm Niçoise-style salmon salad. Also try with trout, cod, halibut and other round fish

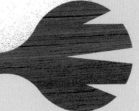

SHELLFISH: SEA FOOD, EAT FOOD

The stars of the classic French fruits de mer, shellfish are just one of the types of edible treasures of the sea. They are naturally ceremonious, sensual and convivial – creating mess, provoking discussion, inducing greed – and fall into two main categories: crustaceans and molluscs.

Crustaceans are like shellfish royalty – with lobsters, crabs, shrimps and prawns reigning – while molluscs can be divided into cephalopods (internal-shelled beasties like cuttlefish), gastropods (with single shells, such as sea snails), and bivalves (with two-hinged shells, like the enduringly popular mussels).

There are of course other less well-known seafood that can't be classified as either, such as sea urchins and sea cucumbers, which are echinoderms. Many are best eaten raw, or cooked with the lightest touch; but, with all as fresh as possible and often should be cooked alive.

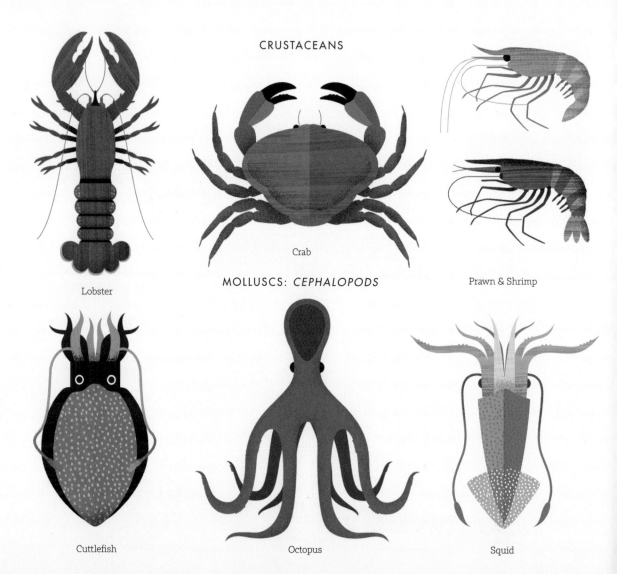

CRUSTACEANS

Crab

Lobster

Prawn & Shrimp

MOLLUSCS: *CEPHALOPODS*

Cuttlefish

Octopus

Squid

MOLLUSCS: *GASTROPOD*

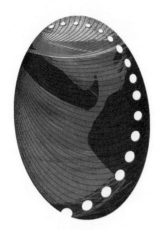

Ormer

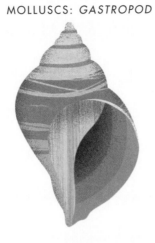

Whelk

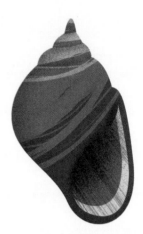

Winkle

MOLLUSCS: *BIVALVE*

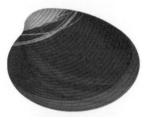

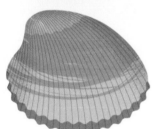

Clam & Cockle

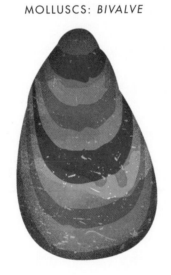

Oyster

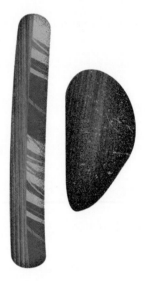

Razor clam & Mussel

ECHINODERMS

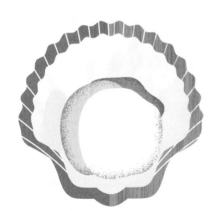

Scallop

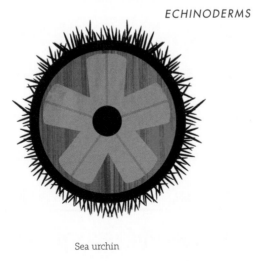

Sea urchin

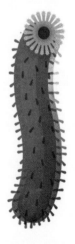

Sea cucumber

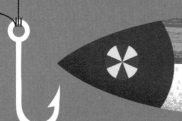

HOOK TO HAND

ATLANTIC SALMON

SOCKEYE SALMON
(Pacific)

CHINOOK SALMON
(Pacific)

CHUM SALMON
(Pacific)

COHO SALMON
(Pacific)

HUMPBACK SALMON
(Pacific)

FARMED

Where fish young are matured in wire cages close to the coast, often in large numbers. Produces fattier, blander fish, and there is much debate about the environmental cost of such intensive practices

WILD

Salmon lay eggs in the gravel beds of streams, which then grow and swim down the river, eventually arriving in the sea where the adult salmon spends up to four years, before starting the process anew

RAW

Super fresh salmon is delicious eaten raw in sashimi or sushi, or dressed in a ceviche

CURED

At its simplest salmon can be cured (changing its texture and flavour) with salt, but often it's a combination of salt and sugar. The Scandinavians are famed for their gravadlax, which combines salt, sugar, dill and white peppercorns

COLD SMOKED

Where cured salmon is smoked at low temperatures (up to 30°C) to preserve and enhance the flavour and texture. Scottish is the best, sliced thinly, and the perfect topper for bagels, rye bread, blinis, and scrambled eggs

COOKED

Baked, barbecued, deep-fried, grilled, poached, pan-fried, roasted, steamed

HOT SMOKED

Hot smoked salmon (up to 80°C) is stronger in flavour and cooked from the heat. It's best flaked in salads, tossed into pasta or nibbled in sandwiches with horseradish sauce

—

SALMON: GO FISH

What once was a luxury foodstuff has now become one of our most eagerly consumed fish across the globe. Salmon – from the Salmonidae, oily family, and so-called 'king of fish' – is loved by humans, bears, birds, fish, otters and seals alike. No wonder, it's a regenerating protein, packed with healthy omega 3 fatty acids and various vitamins, and satisfyingly crowdpleasing in taste. So high is the demand, that we've been farming these marine creatures in the northern hemisphere since the 1960s.

Atlantic salmon is the most popular to eat (praised for its fine flavour), although the five Pacific salmons are currently the much more sustainable option, and can be bought wild, organically farmed, and farmed. Due to the sheer amount we're eating, each has its own issues. As with any animal we're consuming, it's important to be aware of where your salmon has been sourced. Check for sustainable labelling or chat to your fishmonger.

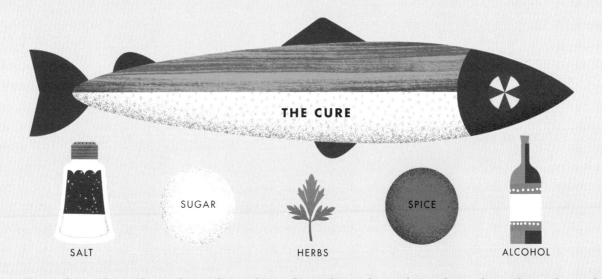

THE CURE

SALT

SUGAR

HERBS

SPICE

ALCOHOL

THE CIRCLE OF LIFE

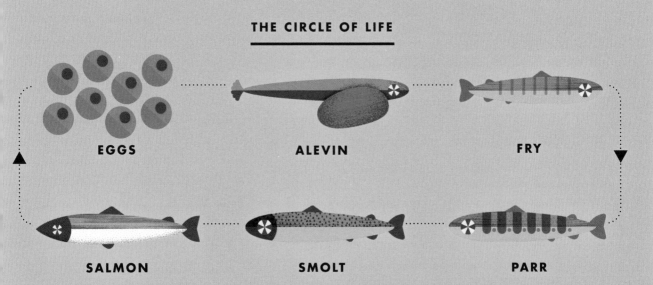

EGGS

ALEVIN

FRY

SALMON

SMOLT

PARR

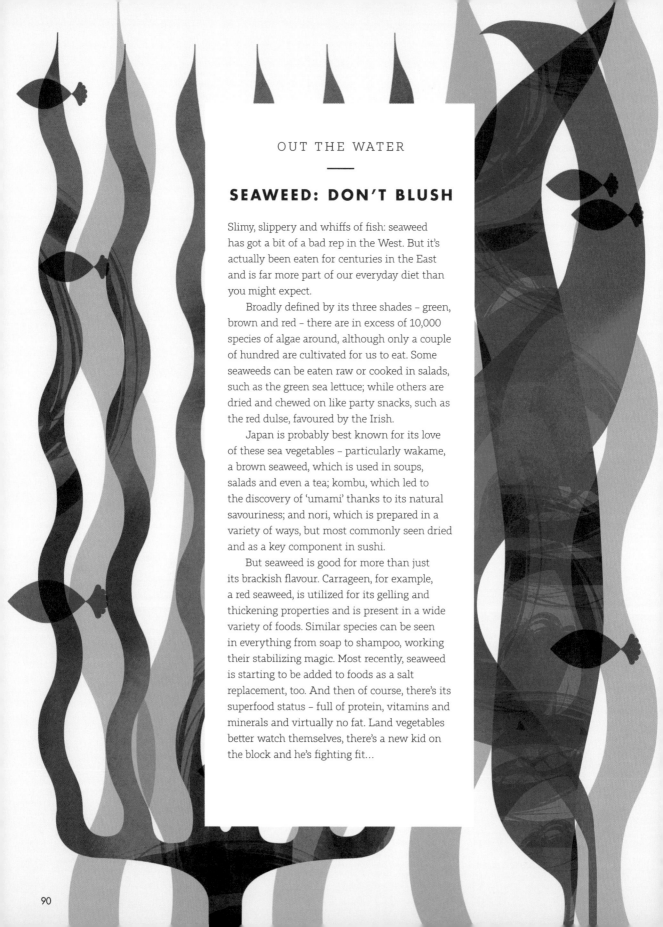

SEAWEED: DON'T BLUSH

Slimy, slippery and whiffs of fish: seaweed has got a bit of a bad rep in the West. But it's actually been eaten for centuries in the East and is far more part of our everyday diet than you might expect.

Broadly defined by its three shades – green, brown and red – there are in excess of 10,000 species of algae around, although only a couple of hundred are cultivated for us to eat. Some seaweeds can be eaten raw or cooked in salads, such as the green sea lettuce; while others are dried and chewed on like party snacks, such as the red dulse, favoured by the Irish.

Japan is probably best known for its love of these sea vegetables – particularly wakame, a brown seaweed, which is used in soups, salads and even a tea; kombu, which led to the discovery of 'umami' thanks to its natural savouriness; and nori, which is prepared in a variety of ways, but most commonly seen dried and as a key component in sushi.

But seaweed is good for more than just its brackish flavour. Carrageen, for example, a red seaweed, is utilized for its gelling and thickening properties and is present in a wide variety of foods. Similar species can be seen in everything from soap to shampoo, working their stabilizing magic. Most recently, seaweed is starting to be added to foods as a salt replacement, too. And then of course, there's its superfood status – full of protein, vitamins and minerals and virtually no fat. Land vegetables better watch themselves, there's a new kid on the block and he's fighting fit…

SO, YOU THINK YOU WANT TO TRY SEAWEED...

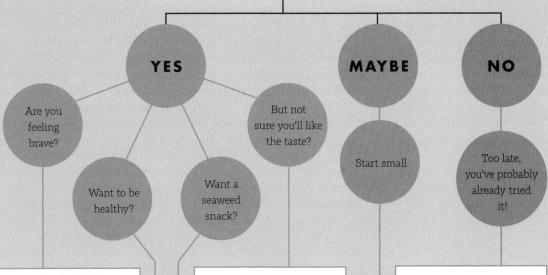

YES

Are you feeling brave?

Want to be healthy?

Want a seaweed snack?

But not sure you'll like the taste?

MAYBE

Start small

NO

Too late, you've probably already tried it!

Try laverbread

Called nori in Japan and sloke in Scotland, in Wales this red seaweed is boiled until it turns to a purée, then made into patties with oatmeal and fried in bacon fat as part of a proper Welsh breakfast fry up

Try norimaki

With sticky rice and fresh seafood and veggie fillings, wrapped in nori sheets, this addictive Japanese sushi is a clean and easy way to incorporate seaweed into your diet

You've eaten jelly!

Some jellies use agar-agar, which is derived naturally from seaweed, as a setting agent and vegan alternative to gelatin, which is sourced from cows or pigs

Try dashi

A Japanese broth packed with nutrients thanks, in no small part, to the presence of brown seaweed, kombu. It's the secret savoury flavour behind authentic miso soup

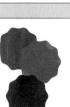

Try seaweed crisps

Brush nori sheets lightly with water, sprinkle with salt and shichimi togarashi, slice and bake at 150°C for 10–15 minutes or until crisp

Try seasoning

From seaweed salts to the Japanese seasoning shichimi togarashi – featuring peppers, roasted orange peel, sesame seeds, ginger and seaweed – can instantly pep up and enhance everything from noodles to beef steak

SWAP SHOP: MAKE YOUR FISHY DISHY GO FURTHER

We're all guilty of it. Whether it be a recipe we cook at home or a dish we order in a restaurant, the food we eat is from a select culinary canon, such creatures of habit we are.

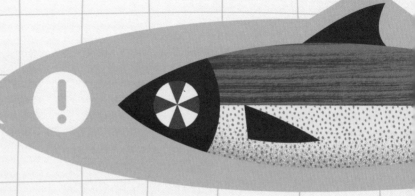

LIKE COD?

TRY TILAPIA

Go spicy and sour in Goan curry

With chillies, coconut milk, garlic, ginger, onion, spices, tamarind, tomatoes

LIKE SMOKED HADDOCK?

TRY SMOKED POLLOCK

Bulk out with rice in kedgeree

With basmati rice, boiled eggs, curry powder, lemon, onion

LIKE PLAICE?

TRY MEGRIM

Go gaga for goujons

Slice into thick strips, coat with flour (seasoned or spiced) and egg (or a thin coating of natural yoghurt), then breadcrumbs, dried couscous, polenta or white sesame seeds. Shallow-fry, deep-fry or bake, and serve between thick slices of white bread, a slather of mayo, lettuce and tomato

LIKE BEEF BURRITOS?

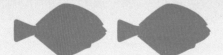

SUBSTITUTE THE MEAT WITH DAB

Experiment with textures in a spicy fish taco

With avocado, coriander leaves, corn tortilla, jalapeños, lime juice, shredded white cabbage, smoky chipotle sauce, sweetcorn, tempura-fried fillets of dab

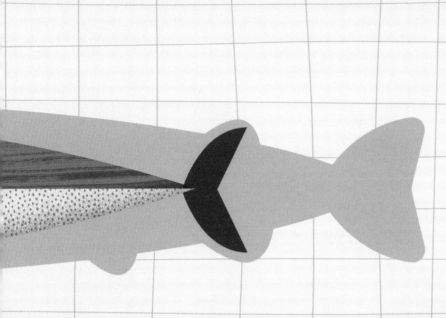

And it's no different when it comes to fish. You need only look at the list of endangered species (from Bluefin tuna to wild Atlantic salmon) to see that we're all eating too much of the same.

So, how about mixing things up and making the most of what we do eat. Bring on the alternatives, try a different flavour, master a new dish. It's time to make the swap…

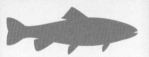

LIKE SALMON?

TRY TROUT

Make it go further with fishcakes

Combine roughly chopped raw trout with crushed cooked new potatoes, lemon juice and herbs. Mould into patties, and shallow-fry until caramelized, and the trout is just cooked

LIKE TUNA?

TRY MACKEREL

Take your salad repertoire up a notch

Dust fillets in flour mixed with Cajun seasoning before pan-frying and serving on a bed of dressed watercress, roasted cumin-dusted chickpeas and orange segments

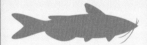

LIKE SAUSAGE CASSEROLE?

TRY CATFISH

Let the fish soak up flavour in a chorizo, catfish and butterbean stew

With butterbeans, chorizo, garlic, onions, paprika, parsley, tinned tomatoes

TAKING STOCK

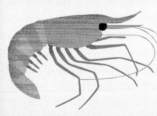

While the idea of fish stock stinking out the house might not appeal to everyone you can make a very speedy shellfish stock that will act like a flavour injection to curries, soups, stews and more. Simply reserve the shells and prawn heads from any recipe that requires prawns. Pan-fry over a high heat with a small amount of rapeseed oil until the little coats of armour turn bright coral/red in colour. Add enough water to cover and crush the shells with the back of a wooden spoon. Bring to the boil and simmer for around 10 minutes. Pour through a sieve, pushing on the shells to maximize the flavour, season, and use your new weapon of mass deliciousness at will!

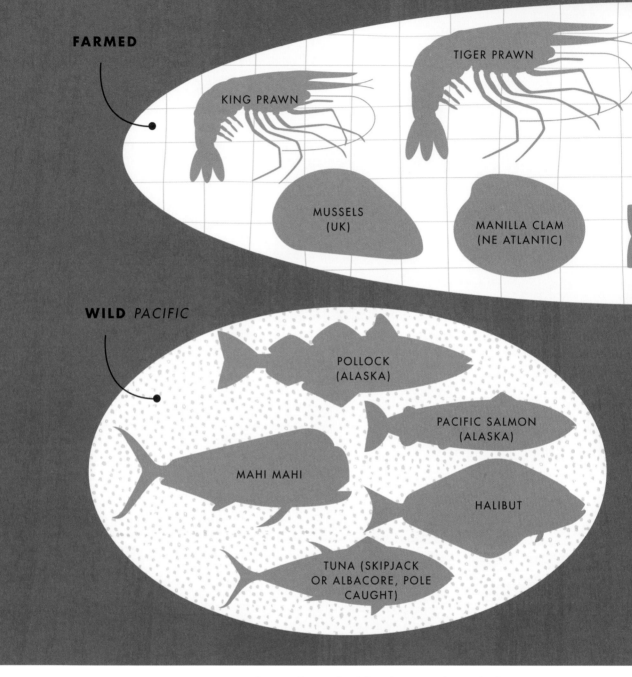

FARMED

KING PRAWN

TIGER PRAWN

MUSSELS
(UK)

MANILLA CLAM
(NE ATLANTIC)

WILD *PACIFIC*

POLLOCK
(ALASKA)

PACIFIC SALMON
(ALASKA)

MAHI MAHI

HALIBUT

TUNA (SKIPJACK
OR ALBACORE, POLE
CAUGHT)

OUT THE WATER

—

SUSTAINABLE: THE YES OR NO GAME

Eating responsibly when it comes to any animal is tough but with aquaculture it's particularly confusing to know what fish and seafood are 'okay' to eat.

While marine farms allow wild stocks to replenish in theory, often wild fish is caught to feed carnivorous farmed fish, such as salmon, which can eat well over three times their own weight. There's also increased risk of disease (and in turn an increase of antibiotics and vaccines being used, polluting the water, nearby ecosystems and fish themselves), and, of course, there are ethical issues to consider with intensive farms, where fish that naturally have whole seas to explore are penned into small spaces.

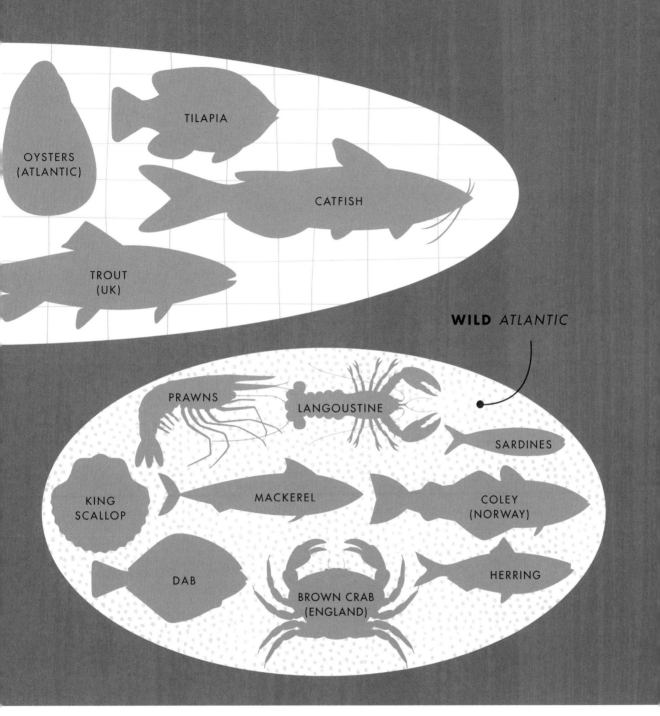

OYSTERS
(ATLANTIC)

TILAPIA

CATFISH

TROUT
(UK)

WILD *ATLANTIC*

PRAWNS

LANGOUSTINE

SARDINES

KING
SCALLOP

MACKEREL

COLEY
(NORWAY)

DAB

BROWN CRAB
(ENGLAND)

HERRING

But with wild fish stocks depleted, devastating environmental damage taking place with trawling and demand ever increasing, what should we be shopping for? Ask your fishmonger about the fisheries it sources from and check for sustainable labelling and certification.

TO EAT/NOT TO EAT

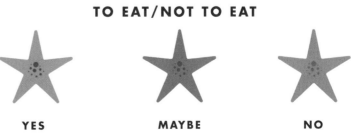

YES   MAYBE   NO

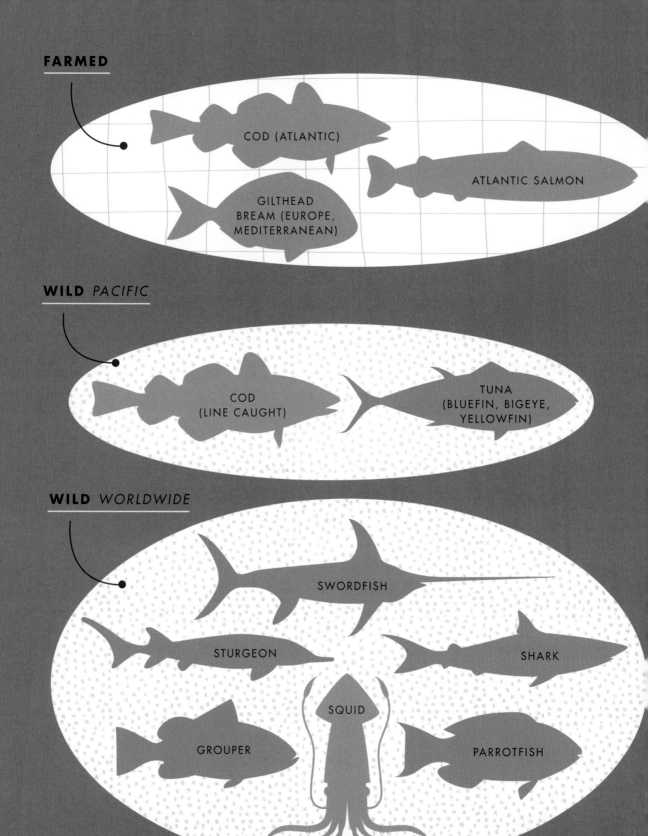

FARMED

COD (ATLANTIC)

GILTHEAD
BREAM (EUROPE,
MEDITERRANEAN)

ATLANTIC SALMON

WILD *PACIFIC*

COD
(LINE CAUGHT)

TUNA
(BLUEFIN, BIGEYE,
YELLOWFIN)

WILD *WORLDWIDE*

SWORDFISH

STURGEON

SHARK

SQUID

GROUPER

PARROTFISH

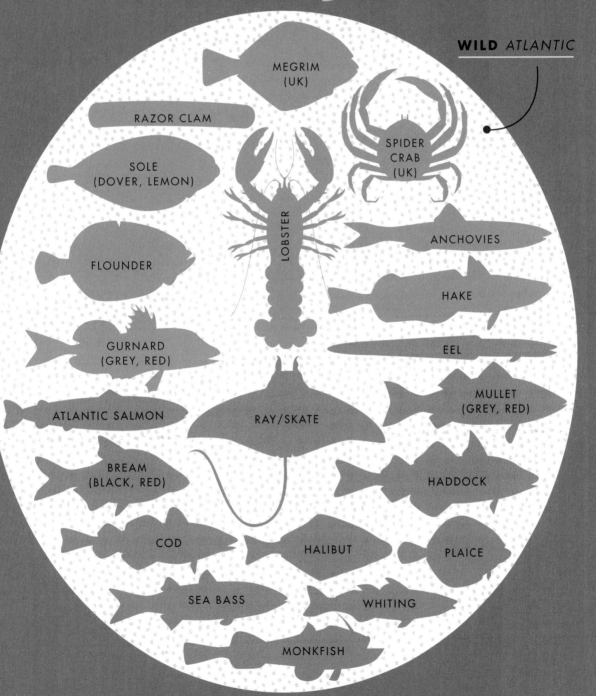

73 MILLION

sharks are killed each year for their fins,
for the Chinese delicacy shark fin soup

WILD *ATLANTIC*

MEGRIM
(UK)

RAZOR CLAM

SPIDER
CRAB
(UK)

SOLE
(DOVER, LEMON)

LOBSTER

ANCHOVIES

FLOUNDER

HAKE

EEL

GURNARD
(GREY, RED)

MULLET
(GREY, RED)

ATLANTIC SALMON

RAY/SKATE

BREAM
(BLACK, RED)

HADDOCK

COD

HALIBUT

PLAICE

SEA BASS

WHITING

MONKFISH

IN THE LARDER

FINE TABLE SALT

The stuff you put in your salt shaker. Often with added iodine and anti-caking agents. Best for baking as it will evenly distribute

HIMALAYAN SALT

Harvested in the foothills of the mountain range. Distinctive pink colour from the amount of minerals it contains. Considered 'pure', it is some of the most expensive salt you can buy

KALA NAMAK

Also known as black salt, although actually pink/grey in colour. Has a strong 'eggy' smell – vegans love the stuff

SEA SALT

Generally larger and coarser crystals. The most famous is fleur de sel from Brittany in France. Great flavour and best as a final seasoning

NOT ALL SALT IS CREATED EQUAL

SEL GRIS

Another French speciality. The natural grey colour is from the minerals absorbed from the clay lining the salt ponds

ALAEA SALT

Hawaiian sea salt that has been mixed with mineral-heavy volcanic clay, giving it a red colour. You can also find hiwa kai, which has added charcoal and a black colour

FLAVOURED SALTS

Salt can be smoked or combined with other flavours such as chilli, herbs, truffle or even vanilla

SALT: OF THE EARTH

Some ingredients we might claim to be 'essential' (chilli sauce, mayonnaise and cheese – preferably all together – being in my top three) but few actually are necessary for us humans to exist; except, that is, for salt.

Whether mined hundreds of metres beneath us and chucked back on to our roads to prevent ice, or hand harvested from the sea and sprinkled in snow-like flakes over our scrambled eggs, salt has the same chemical composition. The sodium and chloride in salt (neither of which we produce naturally) are crucial in sending nerve signals to the brain, muscle function, absorbing nutrients and regulating fluid.

But, of course, aside from its health properties, salt is also vital for enjoying food, too. As one of our five key 'tastes' that we experience (the others being sweet, sour, bitter and umami), salt makes things taste better. From reducing bitterness to enhancing sweetness, it provides balance. It can also be used as a preservative, to improve texture and colour, and as an abrasive. And that's without even touching on the hundreds of ways it can be applied to your beauty or cleaning regimes, or even its powers to ward off evil spirits (a quick pinch chucked over the left shoulder should do it).

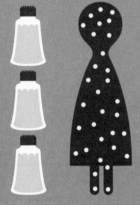

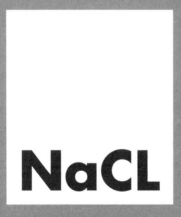

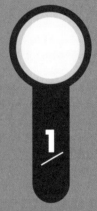

On average we each have approximately 250g salt in our bodies – that's 3-4 salt shakers worth!

Salt contains 40% sodium and 60% chloride

The World Health Organization recommends no more than 5g salt per day (that's just under 1 tsp)

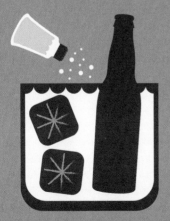

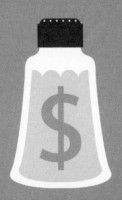

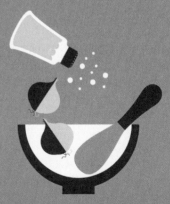

Get beers colder, faster by adding salt to ice water

Salt wasn't always just a seasoning, it was currency too. Roman soldiers used to be paid and slaves bought in salt

Make extra smooth garlic purée by adding a pinch of coarse salt - it acts as an abrasive and seasoning

SUGAR: SWEET ENOUGH?

For something with little flavour and no vitamins, minerals or proteins, it's a wonder that sugar plays such an important part of our daily diets. But thanks to its effectiveness as a sweetener, flavour enhancer, energy source and relative cheapness, it's hard to imagine living without it. Spooned into coffee to give us added pep, sprinkled on fresh fruit, or whipped into fluffy meringues, there are so many different ways we consume it.

While historically we turned to honey, our main source of sugar now comes from sugar cane, which was originally grown in the East before being manipulated around the tropics for commercial agriculture, along with those that grew and harvested it.

The cane is filled with a sweet sappy pulp – the liquid is then extracted and refined, in various stages, to white sugar. Sugar beet, relative of the edible beetroot, which can be grown in more temperate climates, is our second biggest source of the sweet stuff.

Wherever its origins though, highly refined sugar has become the new bad boy of the food world, with nutritionists in their masses calling for avoidance and substitution. It's in part thanks to the rise in consumption of processed foods and fizzy soft drinks, packed with hidden sugars (such as corn syrup) and artificial sweeteners, that many are now turning to alternatives.

THE SWEETEST THING

Sugar cane and sugar beet compete as our top sources of sugar. Cane can be served at various stages of refinement, while beet can only produce refined white sugar

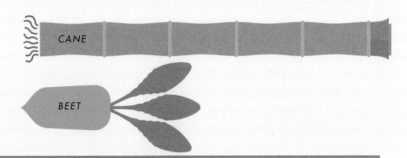

CANE

BEET

Least refined

BLACK MOLASSES
Dark, rich, sticky, almost bitter

DARK BROWN SUGAR
(muscovado)
Moist, fudgy, treacley

DEMERARA SUGAR
Crunchy, butterscotch

LIGHT BROWN SUGAR
Soft, light, caramel

Fully refined

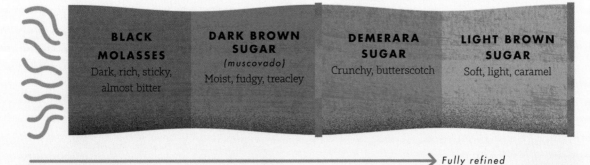

GOLDEN SYRUP
Viscous, light, very sweet

GOLDEN SUGAR
Light, honeyed

WHITE SUGAR
No flavour, sweet

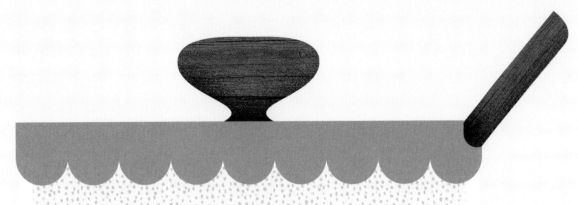

ICING SUGAR
Powdered, the finest of all refined white sugar

CASTER SUGAR
Superfine, ideal for a quick dissolve in baking

GRANULATED SUGAR
Medium-sized crystals, use for crunch or coffee

PRESERVING SUGAR
Large crystals for quick dissolve in jams and marmalades

CANDY CANE

In sugar-growing countries, raw sugar cane is chewed like a sweet

PUMP UP THE VOLUME!

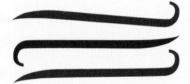

With no real flavour of its own, just sweetness, white sugar is perfect for infusing. Pop a used vanilla pod in a jam jar of sugar for a few weeks and the sweet stuff will take on the spice's heady, ambrosial notes. Other favourites include cardamom pods, cinnamon sticks, lavender buds, lemongrass sticks or thyme

FAIR TRADE FOR A FAIR PRICE

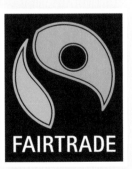

Look out for the Fairtrade symbol to ensure your sugar has been grown and harvested in an ethical way

A WORLD OF UNLEAVENED BREADS

Thought bread meant hours of kneading and proving? Think again. These simple flatbreads from around the world use a variety of flours and are the perfect base for a wide array of toppings

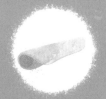

Mexico: Tortilla
masa harina (fine cornmeal), water, salt

China: Shaobing
wheat flour, water, sesame seeds (folded and rolled)

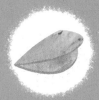

Italy: Piadina
white wheat flour, lard or olive oil, water, salt

India: Roti
wheat flour, water, salt, ghee

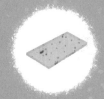

Scandinavia: Rye, wheat and barley crispbreads
various flours, water, salt

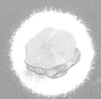

Norway: Flatbrød
wheat/barley flour, salt, sour milk

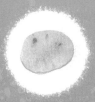

India: Chapati
wholemeal wheat flour, water, salt, ghee

Egypt: Matzo
wheat, barely, rye, spelt or oat flour, water, salt

Norway: Lefse
wheat flour, potato, water, salt

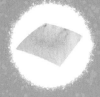

Armenia: Lavash
wheat flour, water, salt, (made paper thin and dried)

USA: Hardtack (or ship's biscuits)
wheat flour, water

Iceland: Flatkaka
rye flour, water, salt

Scotland: Bannocks/oatcakes
oatmeal, butter or bacon fat, water, salt

India: Poppadom
urad or chickpea/gram flour, water, salt, pepper, cumin seeds

THE PROOF ISN'T ALWAYS IN THE PROVE

Want bread fast? Ditch the yeast and look to other agents, such as bicarbonate of soda and an acid, or baking powder, where the rise occurs during the baking, for a shortcut loaf

USA: Biscuit
wheat flour, buttermilk, butter, baking soda, salt

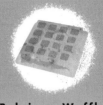

Belgium: Waffle
wheat flour, butter, milk/buttermilk, baking powder, salt, sugar, eggs

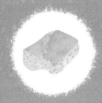

USA: Cornbread
cornmeal, sugar, buttermilk, baking soda, salt

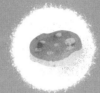

Australia: Puftaloon
wheat flour, baking powder, milk, butter, salt, fried in bacon fat

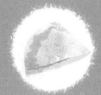

Scotland: Potato farl
potatoes, wheat flour, butter, salt, baking powder

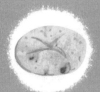

Ireland: Soda bread
wheat flour, buttermilk, baking soda, salt

France: Pain d'épices
wheat /rye flour honey, butter, baking powder, spices

Tibet: Balep korkun
flour, baking powder, water

England: Griddle scone
wheat flour, sugar, buttermilk, butter, baking soda, salt

Serbia/Balkans: Proja
cornmeal, butter/oil, salt, milk/ yoghurt, eggs, baking powder

FLOUR: POWER

The foundation of cakes, the binder of biscuits, the basis of bread; flour is one of our most important ingredients. Essentially a powdery substance created by the grinding of cereal grains (although beans, potatoes, nuts and even some roots can be ground), flour has been used for cooking since the Stone Age.

Before someone thought to add yeast into the mix, flour was combined with water and cooked to make unleavened breads, what we now know as flatbreads. These most simple of breads are made around the world today and an easy, quick and affordable way to bulk out a meal.

50%
of the world's olive oil is produced in Spain

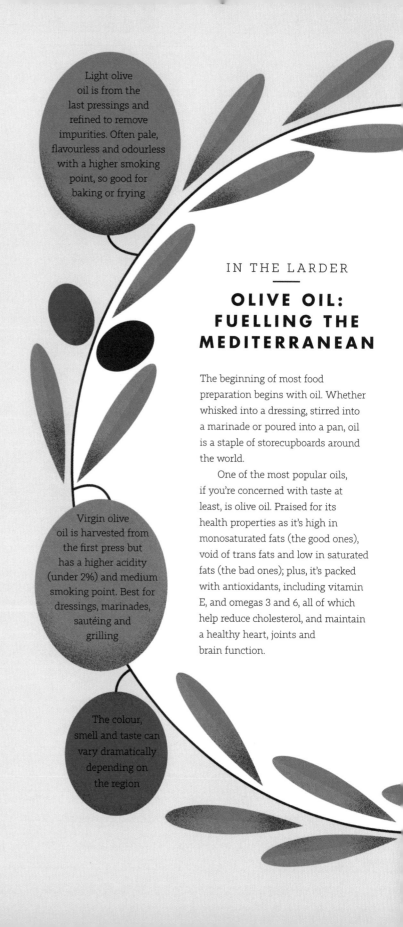

Light olive oil is from the last pressings and refined to remove impurities. Often pale, flavourless and odourless with a higher smoking point, so good for baking or frying

OLIVE OIL: FUELLING THE MEDITERRANEAN

The beginning of most food preparation begins with oil. Whether whisked into a dressing, stirred into a marinade or poured into a pan, oil is a staple of storecupboards around the world.

One of the most popular oils, if you're concerned with taste at least, is olive oil. Praised for its health properties as it's high in monosaturated fats (the good ones), void of trans fats and low in saturated fats (the bad ones); plus, it's packed with antioxidants, including vitamin E, and omegas 3 and 6, all of which help reduce cholesterol, and maintain a healthy heart, joints and brain function.

STORING OLIVE OIL

Air, heat, light and laziness are the enemies of olive oil, so don't be tempted to keep a bottle by the stove, no matter how convenient it is. Corks and screw caps are fine but pouring spouts are not (the oxidization will eventually turn the oil rancid). Keep in a dark, cool place and remember, oils don't get better with age. Buy little and often – keep it fresh!

Virgin olive oil is harvested from the first press but has a higher acidity (under 2%) and medium smoking point. Best for dressings, marinades, sautéing and grilling

The colour, smell and taste can vary dramatically depending on the region

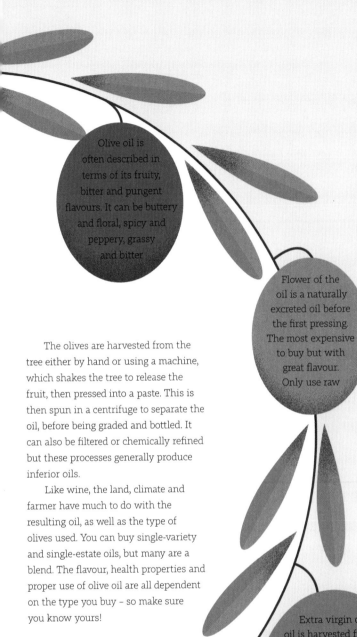

Olive oil is often described in terms of its fruity, bitter and pungent flavours. It can be buttery and floral, spicy and peppery, grassy and bitter

Flower of the oil is a naturally excreted oil before the first pressing. The most expensive to buy but with great flavour. Only use raw

The olives are harvested from the tree either by hand or using a machine, which shakes the tree to release the fruit, then pressed into a paste. This is then spun in a centrifuge to separate the oil, before being graded and bottled. It can also be filtered or chemically refined but these processes generally produce inferior oils.

Like wine, the land, climate and farmer have much to do with the resulting oil, as well as the type of olives used. You can buy single-variety and single-estate oils, but many are a blend. The flavour, health properties and proper use of olive oil are all dependent on the type you buy – so make sure you know yours!

Extra virgin olive oil is harvested from the first cold press of the olives. It is graded on its flavour and acidity (no more than 0.8%). Superior in flavour, aroma and nutrients. Use raw as a dip, in dressings or as a garnish to finish a meal

— **210°C**

OLIVE OIL

— **180°C**

KNOW YOUR SMOKING POINT

Overheating any oil will remove nutrients and destroy flavour. No olive oil, though, should be used for high-temperature deep frying. Try rapeseed, sunflower or vegetable oil instead

24

litres are guzzled per person/year in Greece

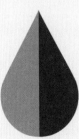

SOY SAUCE: ASIA'S SEASONING

Condiment, seasoning, ingredient, dip, marinade and more – soy sauce is as ubiquitous in East Asian cookery as salt is in the western world. Its recipe is thousands of years old and can come in a number of varieties – thick, thin, light or dark – but is best known for its deeply savoury, almost meaty flavour (despite being completely vegan). If made using traditional methods, it can take a year or more to ferment; while modern interpretations of this natural brew can be nailed in as little as three months. At its quickest though (and most inferior – don't even bother buying it) it can be made in a few days using chemical hydrolysis – where various acids, preservatives, sweeteners and artificial flavourings are added.

SHOP FOR SAUCE

Countries around the Orient brew their own soy sauce – from Japan's rich wheat- (and hence gluten-) free tamari, to Indonesia's thick, dark ketjap manis made from black soya beans. You can even get soy sauces mixed with mushrooms but the two main types to look out for are light and dark. Light sauce is the first press – thinner, saltier and lighter in colour – and best used as a seasoning or in dips. Dark sauce (also called old) is aged for longer, is darker (often with added molasses and cornstarch) and is best used during cooking or for marinades.

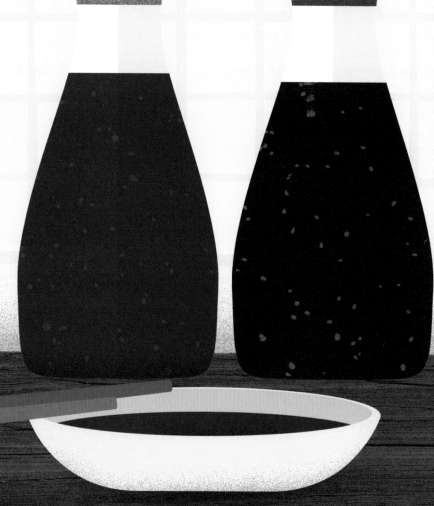

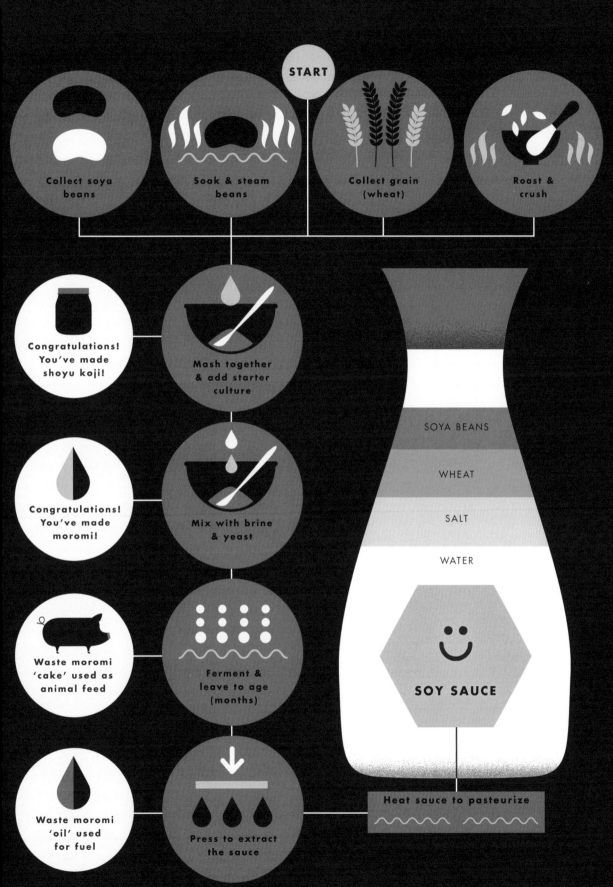

START

Collect soya beans

Soak & steam beans

Collect grain (wheat)

Roast & crush

Congratulations! You've made shoyu koji!

Mash together & add starter culture

Congratulations! You've made moromi!

Mix with brine & yeast

Waste moromi 'cake' used as animal feed

Ferment & leave to age (months)

Waste moromi 'oil' used for fuel

Press to extract the sauce

SOYA BEANS

WHEAT

SALT

WATER

SOY SAUCE

Heat sauce to pasteurize

SAFFRON: THE WORLD'S MOST EXPENSIVE SPICE

The saffron stigmas have been used in cooking, dyes and medicines for thousands of years

The yellow 'male' stamens are of no culinary value

There are thought to be more than 80 types of crocus species but it's only crocus sativus that produces saffron

Each bulb only produces 1 flower

MAKE SURE THE SPICE IS RIGHT

Real saffron will be expensive and its threads will be a deep-red/burnt-orange colour, even in size, and trumpet-like in shape. Good saffron shouldn't contain too much of the yellow stamen (which has no flavour) or rogue petals and will have a floral, slightly metallic aroma. Depending on where the saffron was grown, it should taste mildly honeyed with a touch of bitterness, and should be stored away from direct sunlight. You can buy powdered saffron but only do so from a trusted supplier, as it is much more easily faked or adulterated like this

ISO 3632

The International Standards Organization has its own standard by which saffron is judged, which focuses predominantly on a scientific measurement of crocin (responsible for colour), picrocrocin (the flavour) and safranal (which gives us the aroma). The higher the levels of each, the better the saffron

GOLD

Weight for weight, saffron can be more expensive than gold, making it the most expensive spice on the planet. Luckily, you don't need much to get that golden touch to your dishes – as little as a few strands can be enough. It's better to be cautious than use too much as this super spice can easily overpower

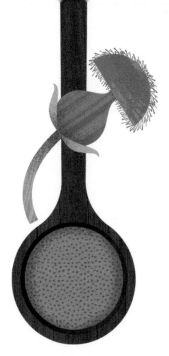

TEA TIME

Unlike other spices, you should never add saffron direct to a dish. It can be lightly toasted and ground in a pestle and mortar, or (best) steeped in a warm liquid such as water, stock or milk, or alcohol, to create an infusion. The longer you leave it (minimum 20 minutes, up to 24 hours) the stronger the flavour

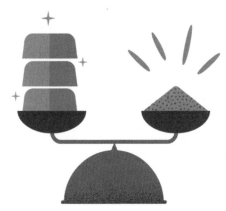

SAFFRON IMPOSTERS

Ersatz saffron has been in distribution for as long as saffron has been sold. Its most common substitutes or adulterers are the yellow safflower (which is also used to make oil) and the spice, turmeric. If it's cheap – it ain't saffron!

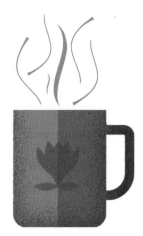

GET COOKING!

Try saffron in some of these classic sweet and savoury dishes from around the world

- ITALIAN RISOTTO ALLA MILANESE
- SPANISH PAELLA
- ENGLISH SAFFRON BUNS
- SWEDISH LUSSEKATTER
- FRENCH BOUILLABAISSE
- IRANIAN CHELOW KABAB

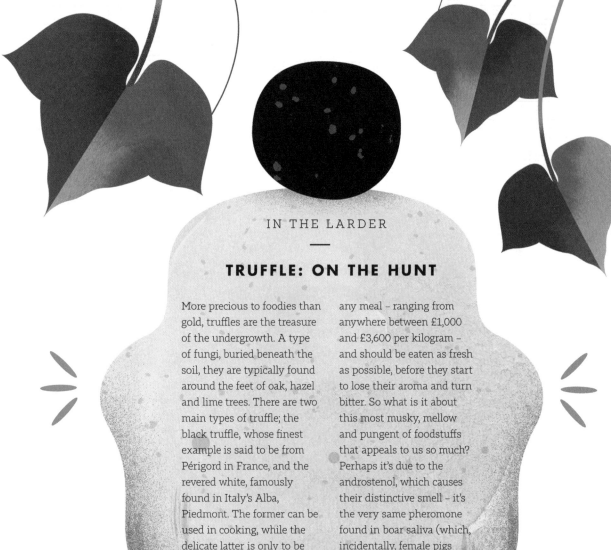

—

TRUFFLE: ON THE HUNT

More precious to foodies than gold, truffles are the treasure of the undergrowth. A type of fungi, buried beneath the soil, they are typically found around the feet of oak, hazel and lime trees. There are two main types of truffle; the black truffle, whose finest example is said to be from Périgord in France, and the revered white, famously found in Italy's Alba, Piedmont. The former can be used in cooking, while the delicate latter is only to be eaten raw, as a garnish.

Either way, they're an expensive addition to any meal – ranging from anywhere between £1,000 and £3,600 per kilogram – and should be eaten as fresh as possible, before they start to lose their aroma and turn bitter. So what is it about this most musky, mellow and pungent of foodstuffs that appeals to us so much? Perhaps it's due to the androstenol, which causes their distinctive smell – it's the very same pheromone found in boar saliva (which, incidentally, female pigs find irresistible) and in the armpits of human men. Go figure.

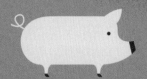

HUNTER GATHERER

Pigs were traditionally used to hunt truffles but they're almost as greedy as us humans, and can't be trusted not to snaffle them on the spot. Dogs are now the hunter of choice during truffle season, which runs from November through to March

PRECIOUS CARGO

The largest white truffle found recently was chanced upon in Umbria, Italy, in 2014 and came in at 1.89kg. It sold for $50,000 (US) at auction – although four years previously a truffle half the size sold for $417,200

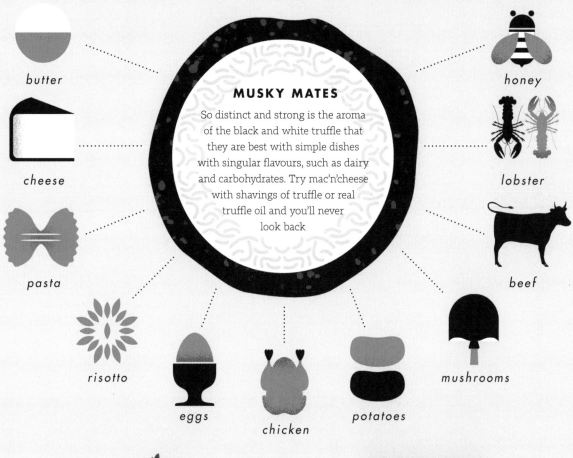

butter

cheese

pasta

MUSKY MATES

So distinct and strong is the aroma of the black and white truffle that they are best with simple dishes with singular flavours, such as dairy and carbohydrates. Try mac'n'cheese with shavings of truffle or real truffle oil and you'll never look back

honey

lobster

beef

risotto

eggs

chicken

potatoes

mushrooms

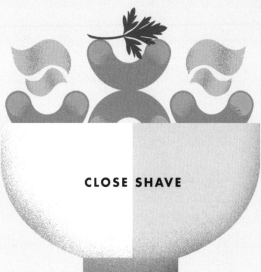

CLOSE SHAVE

Freshly grated or shaved truffle should be used in small quantities or else your supper will taste more like wet socks than a decadent dinner

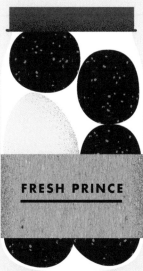

FRESH PRINCE

Fresh truffles should be stored in sealed containers. If you want to make your investment go even further, add a couple of raw eggs to the container and that characteristic musk will penetrate the porous shells ready for a breakfast of kings

RICE: FEED THE WORLD

In terms of human consumption, rice has got to be the most important crop that we grow. It's a staple around the globe – providing food and income for those that need it most. An essential carbohydrate, it provides energy and flavour as the bulk of many dishes. From Indonesia's fried nasi goreng to England's sweet, creamy rice pudding, or China's medicinal porridge-like congee and Spain's seafood-and-saffron-flecked paella.

There are numerous types of rice, and ways to categorize them, but the most useful way of shopping for the grain is to think of it in terms of its purpose. Long grain rice is best boiled or steamed for fragrant individual grains in a Turkish pilaf or a West African jollof,

while medium-grain rice can be stirred into Italy's molten, regional risottos, and glutinous short-grain rice can be moulded into Japan's savoury sushi or pounded into its sweet cake mochi.

Most recipes call for milled, white rice but you can get (the slightly more nutritious) brown rice, as well as black and red rice. Everyone has their own way of cooking the stuff but when it comes to long-grain such as basmati, I always stick to the following rule: double the volume of salted water to rice, boil until the water has evaporated, then remove from the heat, pop a lid on, and allow the rice to steam until fluffy and the rest of your meal is ready. A little knob of butter to finish never hurt anyone.

RICE IS GROWN IN MORE THAN 100 COUNTRIES

3rd MOST PRODUCED CROP IN THE WORLD BEHIND SUGAR CANE AND CORN

158 MILLION HECTARES OF OUR PLANET ARE DEDICATED TO GROWING RICE

RICE IS GROWN IN

- ASIA
- AMERICAS
- AFRICA
- OCEANIA
- EUROPE

WORLD'S TOP 3 RICE PRODUCERS

200M

100M

0M

TONNES

CHINA

INDIA

INDONESIA

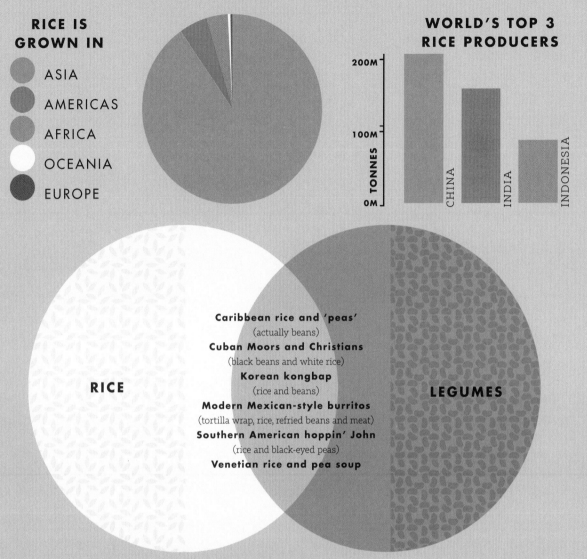

RICE

Caribbean rice and 'peas'
(actually beans)
Cuban Moors and Christians
(black beans and white rice)
Korean kongbap
(rice and beans)
Modern Mexican-style burritos
(tortilla wrap, rice, refried beans and meat)
Southern American hoppin' John
(rice and black-eyed peas)
Venetian rice and pea soup

LEGUMES

MAKE THE MOST OF LEFTOVERS!

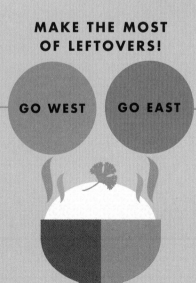

GO WEST

GO EAST

GO WEST

1. Mould leftover arborio risotto into golf-size balls

2. Stuff small cubes of Mozzarella in the centre

3. Dip in flour. Dip in beaten egg yolk. Dip in breadcrumbs

4. Shallow fry in oil until golden

5. Serve with tomato chutney or tomato sauce

GO EAST

1. Leftover basamati/plain long-grain rice

2. Stir-fry chopped spring onions, slices of garlic, ginger and chilli in a very hot wok with flavourless oil. Add the rice, stir fry until heated through and starting to crisp

3. Make a well. Crack in an egg and allow to fry/semi set

4. Break up with chopsticks and incorporate into the rice

5. Finish with fresh coriander

NOODLES: UDON TO CELLOPHANE

How can something so seemingly simple – in its most basic form, just flour and water – be so delicious, and fun to consume at the same time? They're as quick to eat as they are to cook, cheap too, and comforting to boot. They're the fuel of students, the birthday celebration of choice for the Chinese (forget cake!) and the key component to some of the world's most popular dishes. What would pho or ramen be without its noodles?

So, where did noodles come from? The Italians and Arabs might claim it was their original recipe that sparked the popularity but archaeologists would beg to differ, with the discovery of a 4,000-year-old bowl containing perfectly preserved long, thin yellow noodles made of millet flour in northwestern China in 2005.

Nowadays noodles (Asian varieties at least) fall into four main categories – wheat being the most popular (udon, ramen, somen), buckwheat (soba), rice (vermicelli) and egg. They can also be made out of mung beans (that's what makes cellophane noodles so soft and translucent) or even sweet potato (popular in Korea for japchae, where they are stir-fried with vegetables).

They can be flat or fat, thin or long,

1958

The year 'instant noodles' were invented in Japan

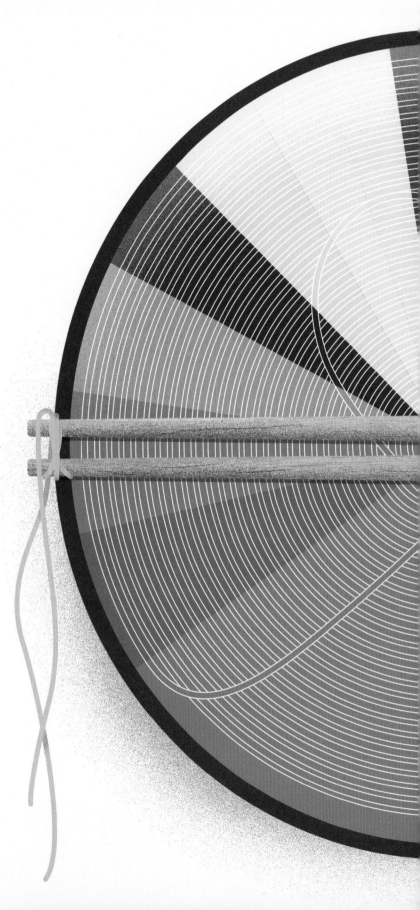

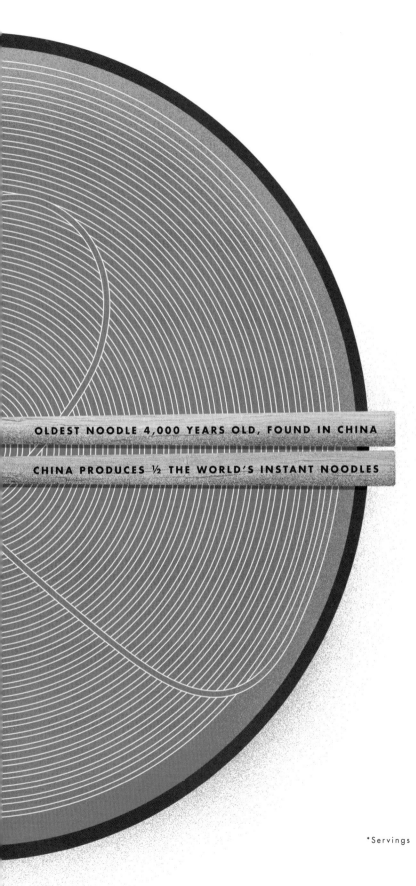

OLDEST NOODLE 4,000 YEARS OLD, FOUND IN CHINA

CHINA PRODUCES ½ THE WORLD'S INSTANT NOODLES

pulled or rolled – with different names, styles and finishes in every country they crop up in. There's even such a thing as a 'rat noodle', named after its short and tapered shape, rather than its ingredients (it's made of rice flour).

They can be as simple as adding water and waiting for two minutes, in the case of instant noodles. The latter is nothing to be sniffed at, either – 105.6 billion bowls of the stuff was served up in 2013 around the world. Most are traditionally eaten with chopsticks (and a spoon if served in a broth) but a fork is more commonly seen in the West.

One thing unifies all of these incarnations though, the way they are eaten – noodles should be slurped, with gusto. Not only does the action cool the noodle down, bringing out the flavours of the dish, but it also shows great appreciation for the chef. And never, ever chop your noodle. Long noodles mean long life and only biting is the acceptable cutting method.

TOP 10 SLUPERS OF INSTANT NOODLES

CHINA 46,220*

INDONESIA 14,900

JAPAN 5,520

VIETNAM 5,200

INDIA 4,980

USA 4,350

KOREA 3,630

THAILAND 3,020

PHILIPPINES 2,720

BRAZIL 2,480

*Servings

PASTA: LASAGNE TO LINGUINE

Pasta can be cooked from fresh (often a combination of 00 flour and eggs), or dried (most often simply durum flour and water) but should always be served 'al dente', literally translated as 'to the tooth'.

The key to cooking pasta is to add your chosen type to a big pan of boiling water – 1 litre per 100g of pasta is the general consensus – with a generous pinch of salt.

SHEETS *Lasagne*

DECORATIVE

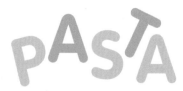

Alfabeto

Fiori

STUFFED

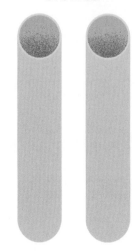

Cannelloni

SMALL

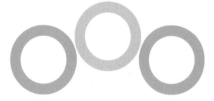

Anellini

Orecchiette

Caramelle

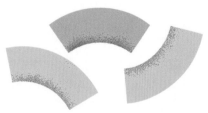

Ditalini

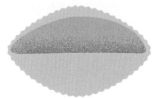

Conchiglie

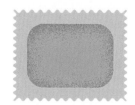

Ravioli

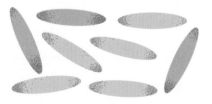

Orzo

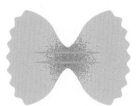

Farfalle

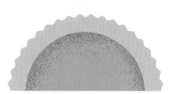

Agnolotti

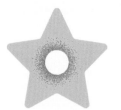

Stelline

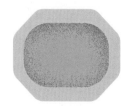

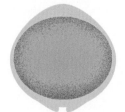

Tortellini

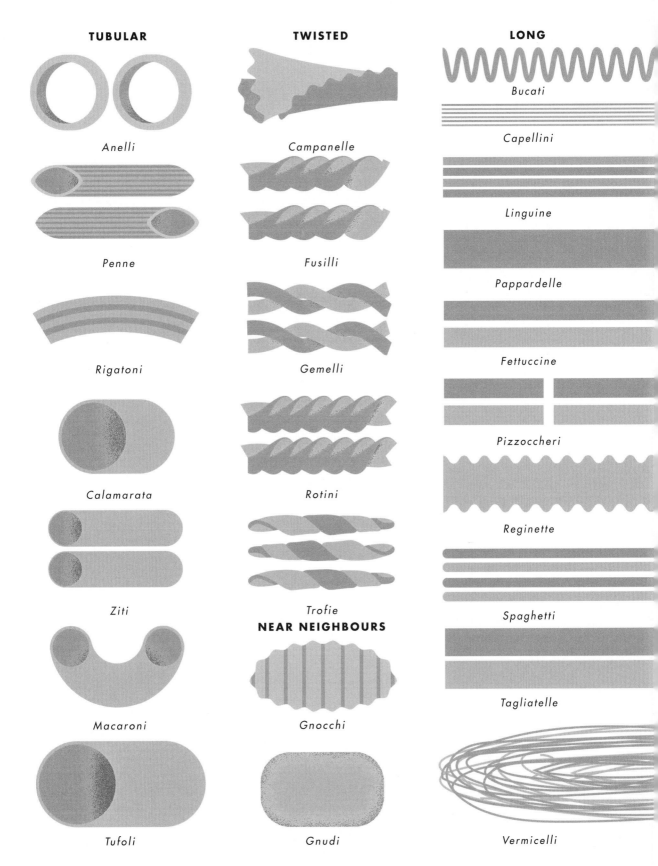

TUBULAR

Anelli

Penne

Rigatoni

Calamarata

Ziti

Macaroni

Tufoli

TWISTED

Campanelle

Fusilli

Gemelli

Rotini

Trofie

NEAR NEIGHBOURS

Gnocchi

Gnudi

LONG

Bucati

Capellini

Linguine

Pappardelle

Fettuccine

Pizzoccheri

Reginette

Spaghetti

Tagliatelle

Vermicelli

TOFU: MINUS THE MEAT

Happy accidents in the kitchen can have delicious results, but for Asia one such 'mistake' has led to the backbone of its cuisine. A staple now for more than 2,000 years, after a Chinese cook happened to curdle soy milk with nigari seaweed, tofu is used in hundreds of dishes across the continent thanks to its bland taste and multiple textures. A blank canvas to allow the region's more punchy flavours to shine, it's since been adopted in the West, too, as a meat-free alternative.

It's also widely touted for its nutritional benefits, which include a high content of B-vitamins and sometimes calcium. And, of course, it's a complete protein source (with some 8g of protein per 100g thanks to its soya bean base) which make it loved by vegetarians and vegans alike.

Tofu is also easy to digest – much easier than the beans themselves – thanks to the fact that the beans' fibrous outer-layers are removed during the manufacturing process along with digestion-inhibiting enzymes. It is also reputed, like all soy-based foods, to lower levels of 'bad' cholesterol. Plus, it is rich in isoflavones, which some say can reduce the risks of osteoporosis, improve menopausal symptoms, and lower the rate of breast and prostate cancer.

BEAN TO BLOCK

1. Dried soya beans are soaked in water for 12-14 hours until they double in size

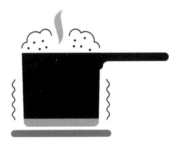

2. The beans are then mashed and mixed with water before being boiled to neutralise enzymes that make them less digestible

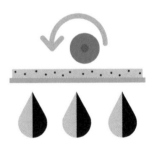

3. Soy milk is extracted with a roller press (leaving the hull and fibre behind), with the remaining pulp reserved for livestock feed

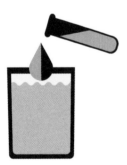

4. A coagulating agent is added to the soy milk to make curds form (similar to cheese making)

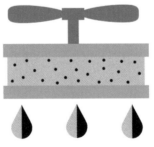

5. The curds are pressed, to squeeze out the last drops of milk, and a large block is formed. (The amount of liquid pressed will determine the final texture of the tofu)

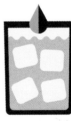

6. The pressed tofu is sliced, washed with fresh water and then pasteurised to make it last

KNOW YOUR TOFU

SILKEN TOFU

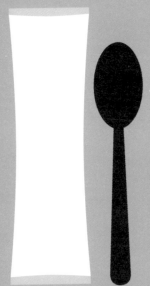

Mositure-rich, silken tofu is undrained, coagulated soy milk that has not been allowed to form distinct curds and has a spoonable consistency. It is often used as a substitute for dairy or eggs in sweet and savoury cooking

REGULAR, MEDIUM AND FIRM TOFU

Lying somewhere in the middle, this tofu has a pliable texture that bounces back easily when pushed with the finger. It can have an outer skin, but a central texture similar to firm custard, making it good for smoothies or blended dishes, or when slightly firmer can be good for stir-fries, curries and more

EXTRA FIRM TOFU

When all the liquid is expelled a very firm block is produced – the Chinese call theirs 'dry tofu'. Rubbery and dense, this is best cubed and stir-fried, baked or grilled, can be crumbled or 'scrambled', and even pickled, smoked and barbecued. This firmest of tofu is also the richest in protein, calcium and vitamins

WHAT'S THAT SMELL?

Just as we preserve our meats and vegetables, historically we've fermented and pickled tofu – making it last longer and changing its flavour in the process. The blocks are air-dried before a slow bacterial fermentation occurs. The fermented tofu is then soaked in salt water, and marinated in various combinations of Chinese wine vinegar, chillies, miso paste or a rice and bean paste; and sometimes red fermented rice is added for colour. The most pungent of them all, though, is known as 'stinky tofu': soft tofu that has been fermented in a vegetable and fish sauce brine. It might smell rotten but to some it's considered a delicacy

THE FLAVOUR SPONGE MYTH

You might think that with its sponge-like texture, that tofu would be good for absorbing other flavours – but you'd be wrong. Unless you have a super-porous type of frozen tofu or a sous-vide machine capable of the six-hour process of completely transfusing the tofu's internal moisture content, you're going to struggle in giving it any significant flavour. So forget marinades, like you'd traditionally do with meats, try glazing instead. Shallow fry the tofu so that it develops a golden, crunchy crust and this will absorb your chosen flavour – from honey, ginger and tamari, to sweet chilli sauce or satay

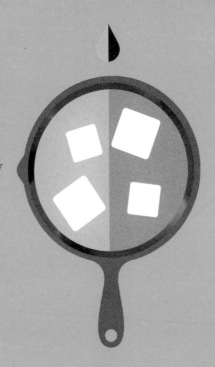

LENTILS: ON THE PULSE

They might be one of our oldest foodstuffs, and a feature in cuisines from Asia to Africa, but in the wrong hands lentils can also be one of our least sexy ingredients.

Its healthy label doesn't help – with one of the biggest protein contents amongst vegetables, just behind soya beans – it's a firm favourite with vegetarians and vegans and has been mistreated in all manner of nut roasts, bean burgers and poorly seasoned soups. But chose the right lentil for the job, cook and season properly, and lentils can be considered perhaps the most versatile ingredient in the storecupboard.

You might be able to get away with tins of chickpeas and certain beans but you should always cook from scratch with lentils if you want to avoid mush. There's really no excuse when they can take as little as 20 minutes to cook: simply place in a pan of cold water, bring to the boil, then reduce to a gentle simmer. Tiny, whole lentils, such as French Puy and Spanish pardina lentils will hold their shape and can be cooked until al dente, while larger or split lentils can be simmered into a creamy purée. Season after cooking, while still warm, with salt and/or spice, and even vinaigrettes.

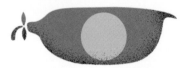

Lentils, like fellow legumes beans, are harvested from pods. Often there are as little as one or two seeds per pod

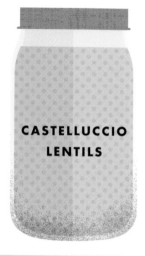

CASTELLUCCIO LENTILS

An Italian lentil, green/brown (and sometimes speckled) in colour, small in size and earthy in flavour. Great in stews and curries, or as an alternative to rice or potatoes

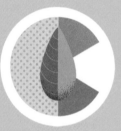

Lentils fried with mirepoix & bay leaves

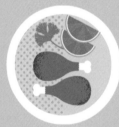

Chicken, blood orange, flat-leaf parsley & lentils in vinaigrette

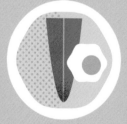

Curried lentils, smoked haddock & poached eggs

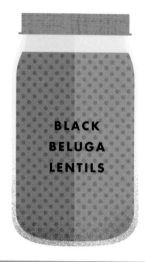

BLACK BELUGA LENTILS

Resembling the caviar of the same name, these shiny black little pearls hold their shape during cooking and are ideal in pilafs and dramatic salads

Roasted peppers, lentils & grilled halloumi

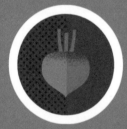

Balsamic-vinegar-roasted beetroot & lentils

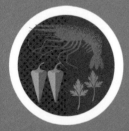

Lime-marinated prawns, red chillies, coriander & lentils

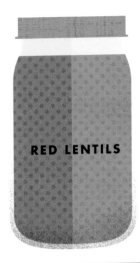

RED LENTILS

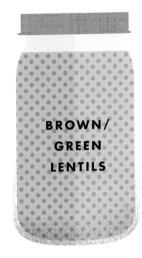

BROWN/ GREEN LENTILS

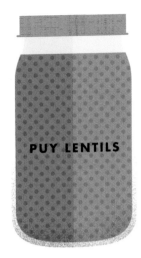

PUY LENTILS

Hulled and split lentils disintegrate into a delicious mash making them ideal for soup, dips and dhal

The larger end of the lentil spectrum, these morsels are an economical filler to soups and casseroles, as they soften during cooking

While most lentils are cheap, Puy is one pricy pulse. Grown in the Auvergne, the beautifully marbled lentils are small, peppery and ideal braised with pork

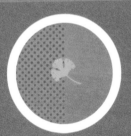

Lentil hummus

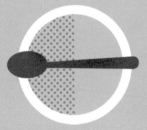

Lentil & vegetable soup

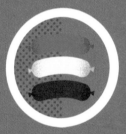

Sausage & lentil stew

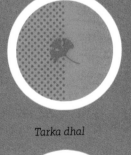

Tarka dhal

Lentil, caramelized onion, bacon & mashed potato

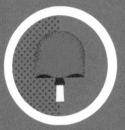

Mushroom & lentil stroganoff

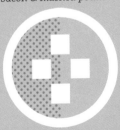

Sambar

Paneer & lentil curry

Lentil salad

THE STARTING POINT

STAY ANOTHER DAY

As well as adding flavour, the lactic acid released by the bacteria as it ferments in sourdough has the added advantage of acting as a kind of preservative, meaning it will last longer

It is possible to begin a starter with just water and flour but live yoghurt will give it a friendly bacterial boost to make sure you achieve a suitably lively sourdough. Be sure to name your starter for best results, and if using a glass jar be careful not to make it airtight, as the wild yeast will release carbon dioxide as it ferments, which could cause a little explosion...

THE INGREDIENTS

50g organic strong white bread flour

50g organic wholegrain rye flour

100ml water (preferably filtered)

1 tsp live yoghurt

THE METHOD

Day 1: In a large bowl mix the flours and water with the yoghurt to form a thick paste. Cover loosely with clingfilm or a tea towel and keep somewhere warm for 24 hours

Days 2-5: Each day add a further 50ml water, 25g strong white flour and 25g rye flour before covering again and returning to a warm spot. A vigorous stir a couple of times each day will introduce more oxygen which will help it get up and running more quickly

Days 4-5: You will see small bubbles forming on the surface of the starter and notice that unmistakable tangy smell. Continue with the flour/water routine

Days 6-7: The starter is now ready to use, but at this point your starter's bacteria need some new flour and water to keep them growing healthily so discard half your sourdough starter and each day refill with 50g rye flour and 100g white flour mixed with 150ml water. Keep in the fridge and it will last indefinitely if well looked after

SOURDOUGH: START SOMETHING

While most bread recipes call for fresh, instant or dried yeast, sourdough (also known as levain bread) requires something altogether wilder. This loaf, with its signature chew and distinctive flavour, uses a wild-yeast 'starter' (which can be as simple as a mixture of water and cereal flour that is left to ferment for around a week) to provoke its rise. The process of making the loaf from start to finish once the starter is cultivated may take as few as 12 hours or more than 24, dependent on the type of flour used, the time of year and even the heat and humidity of the room in which the bread is proving.

Starters can last for decades and in Finland, among other countries, this wild yeast is passed down from generation to generation. Such has been the resurgence in popularity of sourdough cultures around the world, and particularly in Scandinavia, that the Urban Deli in Stockholm now runs a sourdough 'hotel', which will keep starters going while their owners are on holiday.

RAISE A TOAST

Sourdough can take a while to master. The key is a long, slow ferment at a cooler temperature: fast fermentation means the bacteria multiply madly causing a more acidic dough. Frequent 'feeding' of your starter (also known as mother dough) will allow the yeasts to grow into a vigorous starter with the ability to create a good rise in your final loaf. But if you find yourself with a brick-like interior there's always room for toast and croutons!

GO WILD, MAKE FRIENDS

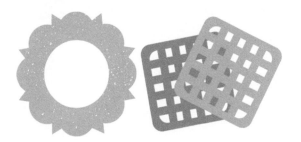

Don't think your starter can only be used for the daily loaf; it can be made into pizza dough, muffins, waffles, pancakes and even cakes, too. Herman the Friendship Cake, for example, is a German tradition where the cake batter is based on a sourdough starter that you feed for several days, then divide and share with friends.

GOING WITH THE GRAIN

It is possible to make sourdough from all cereal grains, although some work better than others. Strong white, hard wheat flour rises most readily because of its high gluten content but if you prefer a whole-grain loaf try mixing half and half wholemeal wheat and white wheat flour or for a rye loaf mix half rye with white wheat. The typically European flavour of pure rye sourdough bread is delicious but rye flour, with its lower gluten content, rises less readily than wheat giving it a denser texture that can be harder to manage.

Some with gluten-sensitivity prefer ancient forms of wheat such as spelt, kamut or einkorn and for those who are unable to eat gluten it is possible make a sourdough from flours such as teff or sorghum.

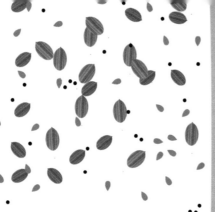

—

BREAD: RESCUING THE STALE

Despite being so ubiquitous, there's not much, actually, that fresh bread is good for (apart from lavishing in butter straight from the oven).
Now stale bread, that's where it's really at. After a few days, when the bread begins to dry and harden, it suddenly becomes the saviour of soups, the prince of puddings and master of mid-week mealtimes. Never let your bread bin be home to waste ever again…

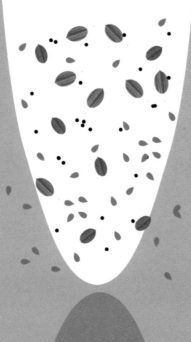

BREADCRUMBS

For 'fresh' breadcrumbs (best with bread a few days old) simply blitz and use immediately or bag and store in the freezer. For dry breadcrumbs, bake the bread until dry and just golden, then blitz and store in a sealed container at room temperature

BINDER
(for sausages, meatballs, veggie burgers and meatloaf)

THICKENER
(of stews and sauces)

SWEET CRUMB TOPPING
(for ice cream or stewed fruit)

SAVOURY CRUMB TOPPING
(for fish, meat, vegetables, pasta, risottos and gratins)

COATING
(for fishcakes, kievs and schnitzels)

FILLER OF STUFFINGS

A MUST FOR SEMMELKNOEDEL
(German dumplings)

NUMEROUS PUDDINGS

SALADS

Crispy croutons or pitta shards are good added for crunch. Start including them in your salads today!

PANZANELLA
(rustic Italian bread, tomatoes, red onions, cucumbers, peppers, basil, olive oil, capers, anchovies, garlic, vinegar)

FATTOUSH
(toasted pitta bread, parsley, mint, tomatoes, cucumber, spring onions, sumac, olive oil)

CAESAR
(toasted bread, romaine lettuce, garlic, olive oil, Parmesan, anchovies)

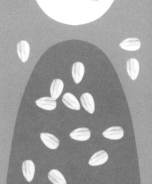

PUDDINGS

Bread works as a great sponge
for flavour in sweet dishes

SUMMER PUDDING
(chilled slices of bread,
soft berries, sugar)

BREAD & BUTTER PUDDING
(baked slices of bread,
custard, sugar)

TREACLE TART
(shortcrust pastry case, golden syrup,
breadcrumbs, lemon)

EXETER PUDDING
(layers of baked breadcrumb-laced
custard, sponge, jam)

APPLE CHARLOTTE
(baked slices of bread, apples,
butter, sugar)

BROWN BREAD ICE CREAM
(spiced)

FRENCH TOAST
(slices of bread, dipped in egg, fried in
butter, dusted with sugar and spice)

BREAD PUDDING
(bread, custard, dried fruits, spice, baked)

BROWN BETTY
(sweet breadcrumbs layered with
stewed fruit)

PANADA
(bread, milk, sugar, nutmeg)

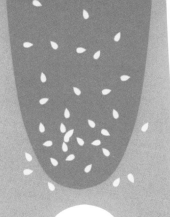

SOUPS

Whether as croutons,
a thickener or a central
ingredient, bread is a great
addition to cold and
hot soups

GAZPACHO
(bread, tomatoes, cucumber,
garlic, served cold)

RIBOLLITA
(bread, beans, vegetables)

PAPPA AL POMODORO
(bread, tomatoes, garlic)

GARBURE
(ham, cabbage,
vegetables, bread)

FRENCH ONION SOUP
(brown onions, topped with a
cheese-laden crouton)

SAUCES

Bread can add a
delicious velvety
texture to sauces

BREAD SAUCE
(milk, cloves, onion, bread,
served with roasted poultry)

ROMESCO SAUCE
(red peppers, paprika,
almonds, garlic,
bread, olive oil,
vinegar)

LAST
CRUMBS

Extra inspiration,
should it be needed

MIGAS
(torn bread, fried with
spices and chorizo)

STRATA
(savoury bread and butter
pudding often with meat or
veg, eggs, cheese)

ANADE
(layered bread casserole with
chard, onions, stock)

**TORTILLA OR PITTA
DIPPING CRISPS**
(sliced, baked in the oven)

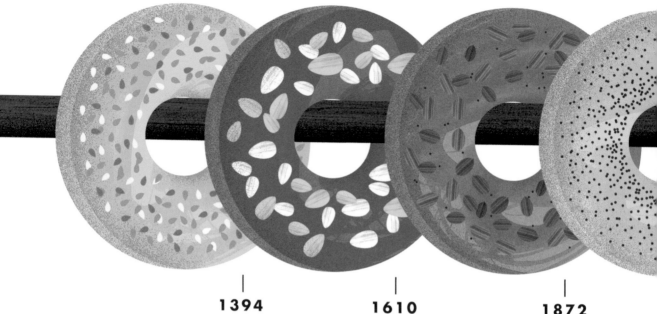

THE HISTORY OF THE NEW YORK BAGEL

1394

First written record of the obwarzanek, in accounts of the Polish royals

1610

First written record of the bagel, in Krakow, Poland

1872

Cream cheese began to be mass produced by American dairyman, William Lawrence

—

BAGELS: THE WHOLE TRUTH

The 'roll with a hole', the bagel has been called many things over the centuries but one thing's for certain, it's special in its form. Unlike most breads, it's boiled before being baked. It only needs a mere flash (often no more than a few minutes) in salted or sweetened water, after being shaped and left to prove at cold temperatures overnight, but it's this that gives the bagel its unique chew and signature shiny crust.

Various stories exist about its origins – some claiming it was a descendent of the German pretzel, others that it was a mutation of the bigger and sweeter Polish obwarzanek – but it first appeared on paper in 1610 in Krakow, where it was recommended that they be given as gifts to women in childbirth. It's distinctive ring shape, with no beginning and no end, is a nod to the cycle of life.

With the migration of the Jews to New York's Lower East Side and London's East End from the 1880s, bagels made their way. It didn't take long for America in particular to adopt the bread as its own, where a New York bagel became a breakfast staple, with cream cheese and lox swiftly becoming the favourite topping.

The bread itself has stayed much the same over the centuries – a combination of flour, yeast, water, salt and malt – although the New Yorkers swear it's their water that makes their bagels taste so good. In Montreal they bake theirs in honeyed water, and modern varieties often contain rogue ingredients – from sweet raisins and cinnamon to cheese and jalapeños. Toppings can vary wildly too – with poppy seeds, sesame seeds, sea salt and crispy onions making an appearance – but you'll forgive me for liking the original best.

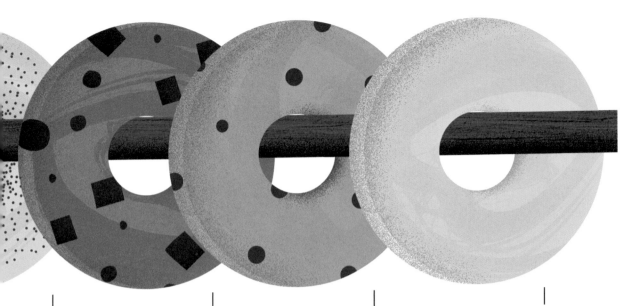

1880

Eastern European Jews, including the Polish, migrated to New York, bringing with them the bagel

1907

The Bagel Bakers Local #338 was formed, with nearly 300 members, dictating the New York bagel market

1960s

New technology enabled mass production of bagels

2008

Bagels made their first journey into space, with Canadian astronaut Gregory Chamitoff

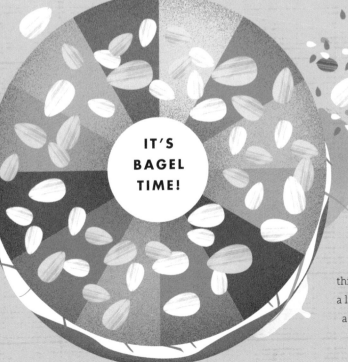

12PM

Lunch – Poppy seed bagel, toasted, with cream cheese, a fold of lox, a slice of red onion, and a sprinkle of capers

IT'S BAGEL TIME!

8AM

Breakfast – Plain bagel, fresh, with crisp rashers of smoky, streaky bacon, a spoon of creamy scrambled eggs and a snip of fresh chives

6PM

Supper – Onion bagel, fresh, with thick slices of salt beef, a layer of Swiss cheese, a heap of sauerkraut, and a dollop of English mustard

PASTRY: FAT CHANCE

Even at its most complicated, pastry is only flour, fat and water (with a pinch of salt or sugar) and it is the starting point for a palmier, profiterole, pain au chocolat and pie; the transformer of frittata to quiche; the crucial element in a croissant and so much more – done well, it is a thing of true buttery beauty. Yet it can go so wrong. It can crumble, it can collapse; it can be tough, it can be the texture of soggy cement, gluing itself mercilessly to the roof of your mouth.

It may have various guises – from shortcrust to choux, pâte sablée to puff – but in the most part the same rules apply. Use the lightest touch and keep it cold. Here are a few others to get you started…

FLOUR

Most pastries including shortcrust, flaky, puff and choux, whether sweet or savoury, need plain white flour

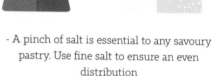

- A pinch of salt is essential to any savoury pastry. Use fine salt to ensure an even distribution
- For sweet shortcrust or pâte sucrée use a tablespoon of icing sugar instead of salt and for further enrichment you can swap the water for egg yolks
- Sweet crusts often turn out better due to sugar making the pastry tenderer as it reduces gluten formation

Butter, as in every other scenario, is best. It will produce the utmost flavour and mouthfeel

Lard (thanks to its lower water content than butter) will produce the flakiest pastry but it lacks butter's flavour

Vegetable shortening and margarine may lack flavour but are a good substitute if you're a vegan

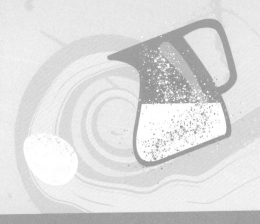

THE MIX

- Liquid, whether water or egg, should be added gradually to achieve a homogenous and solid dough rather than a bowl of crumbs. If it becomes too sticky, cut in a little extra flour with a table knife and draw gently into a ball
- Gluten is the enemy of pastry as it makes it tough. In order to minimise gluten development work dough gently and minimally, just drawing it together rather than kneading it vigorously

THE CHILL

- Keep your cool. Heat is the enemy of pastry: keep ingredients, hands, utensils and work surfaces as cold as possible
- Chilling is essential for two reasons: it allows the fat to harden so that it can properly leaven the pastry when it bakes and it allows the gluten to relax so the pastry doesn't shrink. You can fast-freeze or chill in the fridge for 1 hour
- Suffer from warm hands? Run them under the cold tap before working with the pastry
- Marble rolling pins and worksurfaces are also preferable, as they stay cold

THE ROLL

- Always roll the dough away from you to minimise downward pressure, over rolling and an uneven shape. Roll, turn the pastry; roll, then turn
- Puff pastry is all about rolling and folding. Between each roll and fold, return the pastry to the fridge to chill and allow the butter to harden and help create even flaky layers. And remember, you can't re-roll puff pastry once it's been rolled to shape, as this will affect the rise via the layers of fat you've carefully rolled in
- Always cut pastry with a sharp swift tap of the cutter – no twisting here please, otherwise, once again, you'll affect those layers
- When transferring rolled pastry to a baking tin, drape it over the rolling pin and carefully lift and transfer. It should then naturally fall into place
- Leave some overhang, and trim to fit once cooked to avoid shrinkage during baking

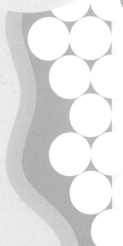

THE BAKE

- Blind baking means pre-baking the pastry before filling it and is advisable if you wish to avoid a soggy bottom. Cover the pastry-lined tin with baking parchment and fill with baking beans or uncooked rice to stop the base rising in the oven: 10 minutes in a preheated oven should do it, then remove the weights and bake for a further 5 minutes until golden
- Egg wash (beaten egg or egg yolk with a splash of milk) brushed over the top or edges of pastry is essential for a glossy, golden finish. Lightly beaten egg white over the base of blind-baked tart cases can also avoid any leakage when adding a liquid filling and cracks are a definite no no!

POWER COUPLES: PAIR THE RIGHT BAR WITH THE RIGHT INGREDIENT

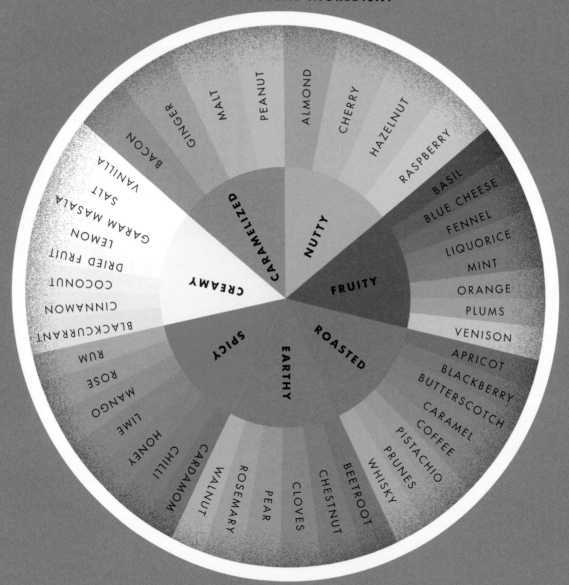

Wheel segments and ingredients:

CARAMELIZED: GINGER, MALT, PEANUT

NUTTY: ALMOND, CHERRY, HAZELNUT

FRUITY: RASPBERRY, BASIL, BLUE CHEESE, FENNEL, LIQUORICE, MINT, ORANGE, PLUMS, VENISON

ROASTED: APRICOT, BLACKBERRY, BUTTERSCOTCH, CARAMEL, COFFEE, PISTACHIO, PRUNES, WHISKY, BEETROOT, CHESTNUT

EARTHY: CLOVES, PEAR, ROSEMARY, WALNUT

SPICY: CARDAMOM, CHILLI, HONEY, LIME, MANGO, ROSE, RUM

CREAMY: BLACKCURRANT, CINNAMON, COCONUT, DRIED FRUIT, LEMON, GARAM MASALA, SALT, VANILLA, BACON

CHOCOLATE: FROM BEAN TO BAR

There aren't many foods that I will admit to sitting on prior to placing in my mouth but chocolate, with its low melting point (some 5°C less than body temperature), seems even more decadent as it begins to soften.

The dark stuff starts life as theobroma cacao, a tree native to the rainforests of Central America. It is cultivated across the globe between 20° north and south of the equator and is as sensitive to its environment and climate, or 'terroir', as wine. Each tree begins producing cacao pods, which can contain anything from 20–40 beans each, after five years.

There are two main crops each year, which are still harvested by hand even now (nearly 4,000 years after it was first discovered by the Olmec people in Mesoamerica), so not to damage the beans, and three main types of cacao that are used to make chocolate.

Forastero is what you'll find in most bars; Criollo is typically low-yielding and as a result rarely seen (it accounts for around 5% of global production); while Trinitario is a hybrid between the two. Each has its own distinctive flavour but the taste (whether it be fruity and floral, or nutty and spicy) of the finished chocolate will be dependent on the cacao variety, where it was grown and how it was processed.

When it comes to enjoying the 'food of the gods', you should use all of your senses. Start by looking at the chocolate, then smell and take in the aromas. Bend the bar to listen for a good, clean snap; then place a piece on your tongue and let it melt. Place another piece in your mouth (okay, and another) and chew to enjoy all the layers of flavour (there are 100s to detect, once you become a pro).

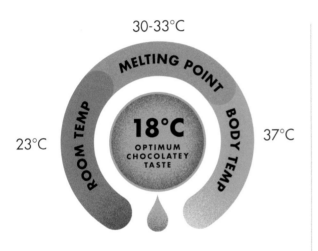

30-33°C

MELTING POINT

ROOM TEMP

23°C

18°C
OPTIMUM
CHOCOLATEY
TASTE

BODY TEMP

37°C

TANNIN TANTRUM

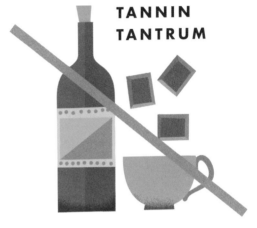

Avoid red wine (unless sweet) and black tea with dark chocolate as all three have drying tannins!

THE JOURNEY

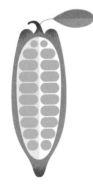

1. Pods are harvested by hand and cracked open using a stick. The outer husk is then used for compost, animal feed or soap making

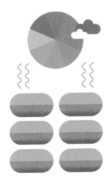

2. Beans, still covered in their sweet, edible pulp are left to ferment in the natural heat for up to seven days

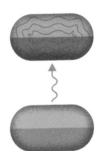

3. They are then spread out and left to dry until nearly all the moisture disappears

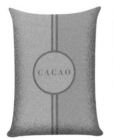

CACAO

4. The beans are graded, bagged and shipped, before being cleaned of unwanted extras such as stones

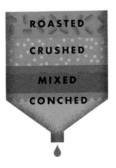

ROASTED

CRUSHED

MIXED

CONCHED

5. Beans are roasted and cracked to reveal cocoa nibs. Nibs are ground to create cocoa liquor and mixed with sugar, extra cocoa butter, milk, vanilla and emulsifiers

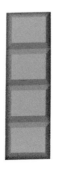

6. The chocolate is then conched (kneaded and smoothed), tempered (heated and cooled) and moulded into bars and left to cool and set

ICE CREAM: ICE, ICE BABY

Is there any sweeter sound than that of the tinny music played from an ice-cream van? The answer is no and that's because ice cream is a thing of true culinary beauty. Frozen cream: ambrosial, comforting and decadent, it can even mend broken hearts.

Rumours abound about its origins – Alexander the Great is said to have enjoyed snow flavoured with honey and nectar and Roman emperor Nero made the most of his slaves by sending them up mountains to collect snow that was destined to be combined with fruit and their juices – but the lady who we really owe our sweet love affair to is the Italian-born French royal, Catherine de Medici. Her love of fine foods in the mid-1500s transformed French gastronomy and ice cream was one of many dishes Catherine and her chefs introduced to the country.

Back then, of course, before freezers existed, ice cream was made using salt and ice (the former brings the temperature down to below freezing – a good trick for keeping your beers cool, too!). These days though, ice cream can be made almost instantly with liquid nitrogen and even via a 3D printer.

So, what's in ice cream? Cream, naturally, and sometimes milk, sugar and often eggs. But there's also a crucial invisible ingredient – air. Whether beaten in before freezing (some recipes call for a base of Italian meringue, or in the instance of parfait, a mousse of egg yolks and sugar) or during the freezing process through churning, air is what makes ice cream so moreishly creamy and light.

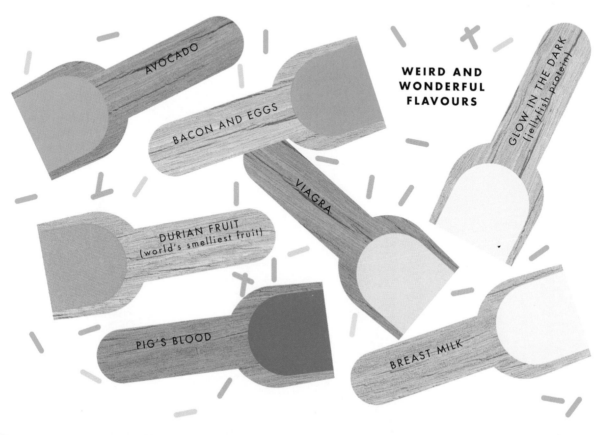

WEIRD AND WONDERFUL FLAVOURS

AVOCADO

BACON AND EGGS

GLOW IN THE DARK (jellyfish protein)

VIAGRA

DURIAN FRUIT (world's smelliest fruit)

PIG'S BLOOD

BREAST MILK

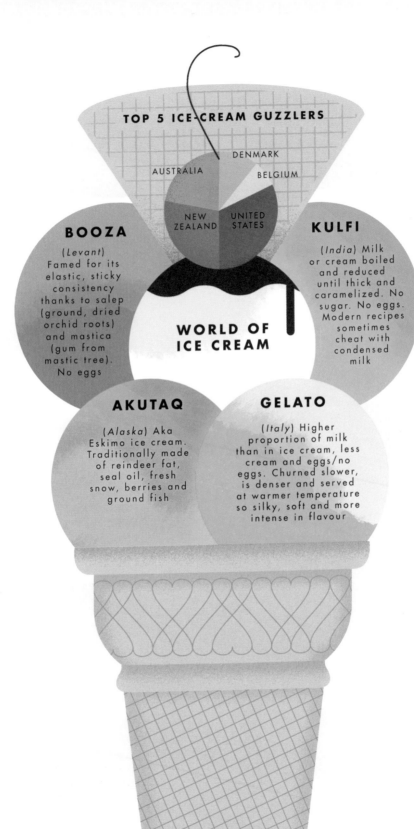

TOP 5 ICE-CREAM GUZZLERS

AUSTRALIA

DENMARK

BELGIUM

NEW ZEALAND

UNITED STATES

BOOZA

(*Levant*) Famed for its elastic, sticky consistency thanks to salep (ground, dried orchid roots) and mastica (gum from mastic tree). No eggs

KULFI

(*India*) Milk or cream boiled and reduced until thick and caramelized. No sugar. No eggs. Modern recipes sometimes cheat with condensed milk

WORLD OF ICE CREAM

AKUTAQ

(*Alaska*) Aka Eskimo ice cream. Traditionally made of reindeer fat, seal oil, fresh snow, berries and ground fish

GELATO

(*Italy*) Higher proportion of milk than in ice cream, less cream and eggs/no eggs. Churned slower, is denser and served at warmer temperature so silky, soft and more intense in flavour

JAM: HOT

It might be hard to believe but this everyday spread actually has ancient relatives. Ripe fruit was packed in containers with honey to preserve it – quince was a favourite, and called melomeli by the Greeks – but it wasn't until the introduction of cane sugar that jam as we know it was made.

Traditional schools of thought suggest that the perfect jam needs equal weight of sugar to fruit – that's to get the right ratio of jam's three essential ingredients, sugar, pectin and acid – but cooks continue to experiment. Understanding the science though is fundamental to the finished product.

Fruit is boiled to release the pectin – it's this that will eventually help to set the fruit in its sweet syrup. Pectin molecules form in chains that function almost like a net, bringing everything together. Water isn't pectin's friend, and it's the sugar that helps to bind the water, allowing pectin to work unthwarted. Pectin also has a slight negative charge, which is dealt with by the acid naturally occuring in the fruit, or is added via lemon juice. Pectin happy, the fruit and sugar gel, and your jam is made.

1 KG

1 KG

½ LEMON

0.5% PECTIN

60% SUGAR

PICK THE RIGHT FRUIT

If you're cooking with a low pectin fruit it's a good idea to throw in some high pectin fruit, too, to give everything a helping hand

HIGH	LOW
quince	apricots
apples	rhubarb
blackberries	strawberries
lemon	blueberries
pear	cherries
oranges	peaches
gooseberries	pineapple
plums	raspberries
grapes	bananas
cranberries	melons

GAME, SET, SERVE

Before jam was slathered on toast or between cake sponges, it was often served as a treat on teaspoons alongside tea and this ritual is still practiced now in certain regions including Greece, Cyprus, Turkey, Iran and much of the Middle East

TOP TIPS

- Choose only under ripe and/or just ripe fruit – anything 'over' will have less pectin and produce an inferior spread
- Make sure you are using the right sugar for the recipe: 'jam' sugar will contain extra pectin and could cause a stiff jam if used when not required
- Macerating fruits (strawberries and tomatoes work well with this method) overnight in sugar is a great way to kickstart your jam
- Make sure all of the sugar is dissolved before bringing it to the boil or you risk a caramelized flavour or crystallisation
- Once you've mastered a basic fruit jam experiment with additional flavours – perhaps raspberry and rose, gooseberry and elderflower, damson and vanilla, or rhubarb and ginger
- You can skim off the scum that forms on the surface of the jam using a spoon or add a small knob of butter to help it disperse
- Allow the jam to rest for 5-10 minutes after removing from the heat before pouring into jars to ensure an even distribution of fruit
- Keep stirring to a minimum

CLEAN BANDIT

Cleanliness is essential during jam making. Sterilise jars before filling: this can be done by washing and rinsing the jars before 'drying' in an oven at 140°C or by placing on a hot wash in the dishwasher. Both the jar and jam should still be warm when bottling, the jam should then be sealed with a wax paper disc, and topped with a lid. Add dated labels to the jars once cool

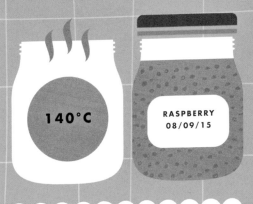

140°C

RASPBERRY 08/09/15

SWEET Vs SAVOURY

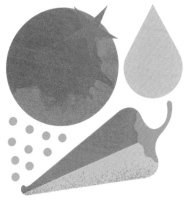

Jam doesn't just have to be sweet – savoury jams work on the same principles. You can either add savoury elements to fruit, be it herbs or spices, or you can take traditionally savoury ingredients, such as tomatoes, peppers, chillies or even bacon and combine with sugar or syrups

WRINKLE TEST

With pectin varying from fruit to fruit, and even with the fruit's ripeness, timings for that 'perfect' set are hard to judge. At the start of any preserving, place some plates in the freezer. When you think the jam is ready, spoon a small amount on to the chilled plate. Allow the jam to cool for a few minutes, then push the jam back with your finger. When 'set' it should wrinkle, if not, place the pan back on the heat and continue to boil for a few more minutes, then test again. Repeat until necessary

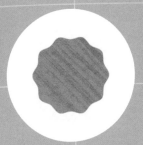

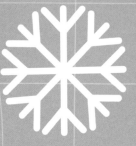

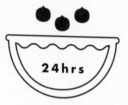

1. Soak chickpeas

200g dried chickpeas

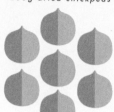

2. Drain

1/2 tsp bicarbonate of soda

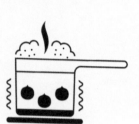

3. Bring chickpeas with soda to the boil, and simmer for 30 minutes or until soft

2 finely grated garlic cloves

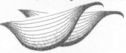

4. Drain, allow to cool and reserve 1/2 a cup of water

juice of 1 lemon

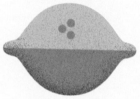

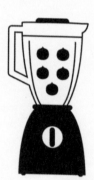

5. Blitz chickpeas

2 tbsp tahini

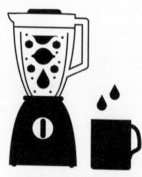

6. Add garlic, lemon, tahini and salt and blitz with enough cooled liquid until smooth

large pinch of salt

7. Pour into a bowl and swirl with the back of a spoon

drizzle of oil

8. Drizzle with olive oil. Serve at room temperature

HUMMUS RECIPE

HUMMUS: THE DIP THAT TRANSCENDS RELIGION AND INTERNATIONAL BOUNDARIES

When swirled around its chosen vessel, drizzled with deep green olive oil into luxurious pools, and flecked with a scarlet dust of smoked paprika, hummus is edible proof that we eat with our eyes as much as our mouth. A little careful consideration and this modern storecupboard staple is a transcendental dip.

An ancient Levantine speciality, this is a dish that makes the humble chickpea, a hero. Blitzed with garlic, tahini (sesame seed paste), salt and lemon juice, these protein-packed legumes suddenly become a creamy invitation for everything from toasty shards of pitta bread or crunchy crudités, to its spiritual brother, the falafel.

As with anything this simple, ingredients are key. If you want a superior hummus, you'll shun tinned or jarred chickpeas in favour of soaking and cooking your own from dry. And be sure to find a decent tahini, or else you'll hear cries of 'pass the tzatziki'.

ADD TO THE BLENDER:

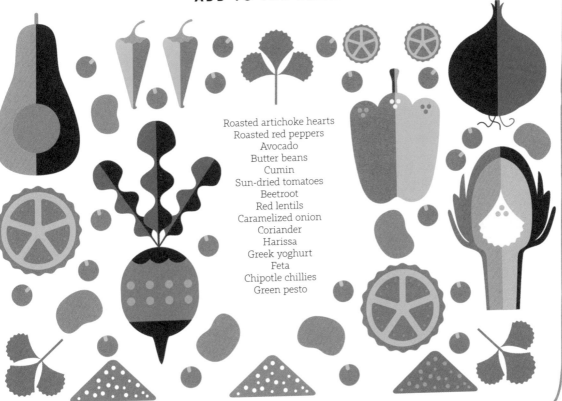

Roasted artichoke hearts
Roasted red peppers
Avocado
Butter beans
Cumin
Sun-dried tomatoes
Beetroot
Red lentils
Caramelized onion
Coriander
Harissa
Greek yoghurt
Feta
Chipotle chillies
Green pesto

VINAIGRETTE: IT'S ALL IN THE BALANCE

EXTRAS

Like it creamy? Bind in a little crème fraîche. Like it cheesy? Blend with Roquefort or Dolcelatte

OIL

Extra virgin olive or rapeseed oil is ideal, although nut, sesame and hemp oils can also work. You want something with a flavour of its own, so leave the tasteless oils for the fryer

VINEGAR

Avoid harsh malt vinegar (save that for your chips), try white and red wine vinegars; sherry, cider, balsamic or rice vinegars; or lemon or lime juice (although you might need more of the latter)

Picked straight from the ground, untouched by seasoning or dressing, it's hardly surprising that lettuce leaves get a bad name – discarded by the more foolish foodie as 'rabbit food'. Even a simple drizzle of grassy olive oil and a few flakes of sea salt can lift a leaf. But treat a salad to a proper dressing and you've got yourself a masterful meal.

Because it is so basic, only the best ingredients will do. Layer the ingredients in a jam jar – seasonings first, then vinegar and oil – and shake it (lid on) until the mix is completely emulsified.

Leaves should always be dressed last minute, and sparingly, to minimize wilting – while sturdier salad items, such as tomatoes, cucumber, avocado, artichoke hearts, asparagus or courgettes et al, can take it (and actually get better) earlier. Vinaigrette can also be used to dress hot items, too – think new potatoes, beans (green, butter or broad), roasted peppers, and blanched spring/early summer veg (purple sprouting broccoli, peas, kale).

SEASONING

Salt and pepper is essential but you can also add mustard (Dijon, English or wholegrain), grated horseradish or wasabi, soy or fish sauce, finely chopped fresh herbs, sliced red chillies, minced garlic, finely diced shallot, finely chopped anchovies, honey, and/or fried bacon, depending on the dressing's final destination

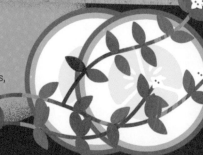

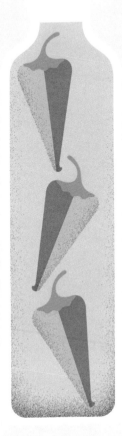

SPEED THINGS UP

Add instant flavour to vinaigrettes with infused olive or rapeseed oils – just make sure your chosen ingredient is always covered by the oil while it's infusing

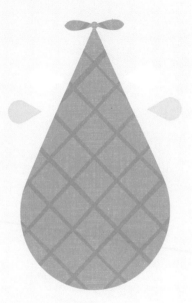

YOU SPIN ME RIGHT ROUND

Wash salad leaves by gently swilling in a sink full of cold water, then dry thoroughly before dressing to ensure an even coating. This can be done in a salad spinner, or place the drained leaves in a clean tea towel. Bring all four corners of the tea towel together, hold tightly and swing with wild abandon (well, not too much abandon…)

LOVE ME TENDER

Vinaigrettes can also work well as a marinade (and tenderizer) for meats, fish and veg before grilling – this works especially well with dressings that include strong flavours such as balsamic vinegar, rapeseed oil, honey and hot mustard; or rice wine vinegar with toasted sesame oil, freshly minced ginger and dark soy sauce

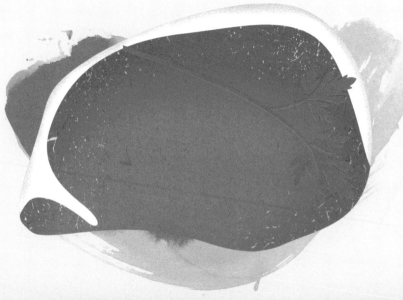

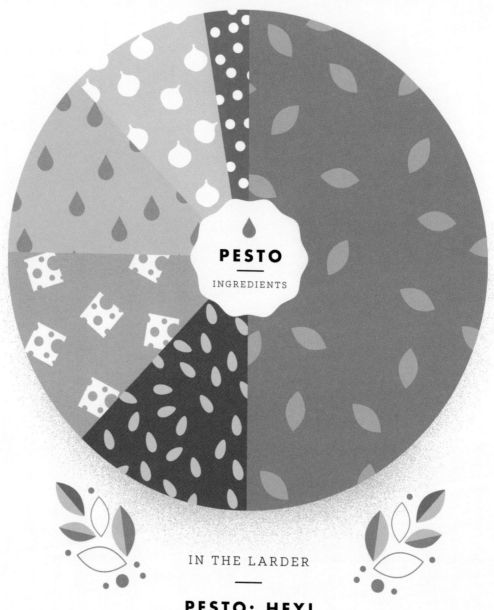

PESTO

INGREDIENTS

IN THE LARDER

—

PESTO: HEY!

Just as Bologna has its ragu and Naples its pizza, the port of Genoa in northern Italy has pesto. Featuring, at its most authentic, only six ingredients and with no cooking involved, it is hardly surprising that this simple sauce now pops up in dishes around the world.

There are debates about whether the raw condiment originated with the Romans, Persians or Arabs, with various evolutions of herb and garlic combinations cropping up throughout the ages, but the first recipe in the form we know it today was recorded in the 19th century.

The star of pesto, of course, is basil – a soft, green,

sweet and slightly aniseedy herb. It's the leaves you need, and young ones at that – no stalk and definitely not dried – or you can blanch the older ones for 30 seconds before plunging into ice water, to remove some of the bitterness. The garlic, too, should be young, fresh and juicy when crushed. Pine nuts should be European (Chinese pine nuts can sometimes cause the highly unpleasant 'pine mouth', which causes a bitter taste that lasts for weeks) and untoasted; while the olive oil, which binds it all together, should be good quality but light and neither too peppery nor grassy. Traditionally, hard and salty Italian cheese is used, such as Pecorino or Parmesan (or often a combination of the two). And coarse sea salt is as important as a seasoning as an abrasive.

The way and order they are combined is crucial. Purists dictate that a wooden pestle and marble mortar should be used, to gently grind the ingredients together (first the garlic and nuts, next the basil and salt, before finally trickling in the oil, and stirring in the grated cheese) but modern cooks (let's just call them cheats) ask for a food processor and the odd push of the pulse button.

In Genoa you'll find the sauce bound through trofie pasta (which is short, thin and twisted) or stirred into trenette (similar to linguine) with cooked potatoes and green beans. It's also popular layered in lasagne, thrown into gnocchi and as a garnish for soup; as well as a million other contemporary uses (think sandwich filler, crudité dipper, and more). So well loved and valued is the recipe to the Ligurian region that there is even now an Order of the Pesto Brotherhood to help protect and promote the authentic sauce.

INGREDIENT KEY

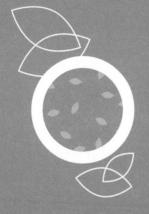

Basil
(young leaves)

Alternatives – coriander, mint, nettles, oregano, parsley, pea shoots, rocket, sorrel, watercress, wild garlic; or you can go really wild with roasted red bell peppers or sun-dried tomatoes

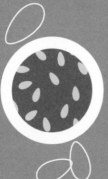

Pine nuts
(European)
Alternatives – almonds, cashews, cob nuts, hazelnuts, macadamia, pistachios, peanuts, sunflower seeds (toasted), walnuts

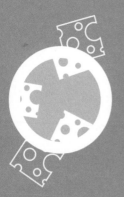

Cheese
(Parmesan)
Alternatives – any hard, aged salty cheese will work well such as Pecorino, mature Cheddar, Grana Padano or Manchego

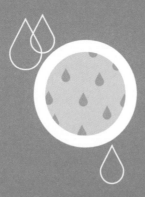

Olive oil
(a light and fruity extra virgin)

Alternatives – avoid overly grassy or peppery oils as this will overpower the sauce. Try rapeseed oil or melted butter

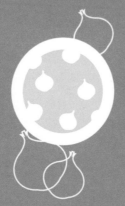

Garlic
(young, fresh without any green shoots)

Alternatives – some recipes avoid the strong flavour of garlic altogether, so you could use chives or wild garlic instead

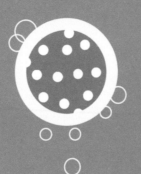

Salt
(coarse sea salt)

Alternatives – you don't need much as the cheese is salty but coarse salt is essential as an abrasive to help break the ingredients down into a silky sauce. Experiment with flavoured salts

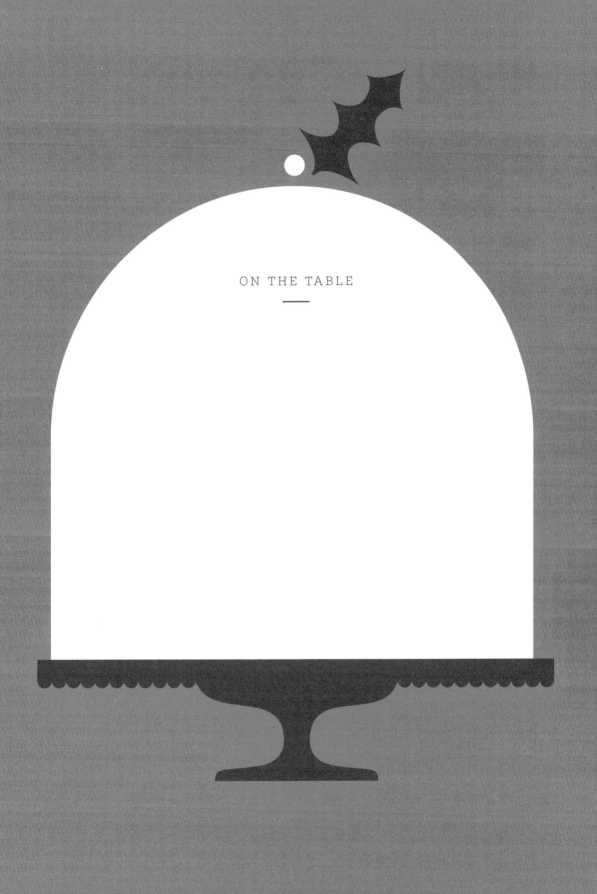

ON THE TABLE
—

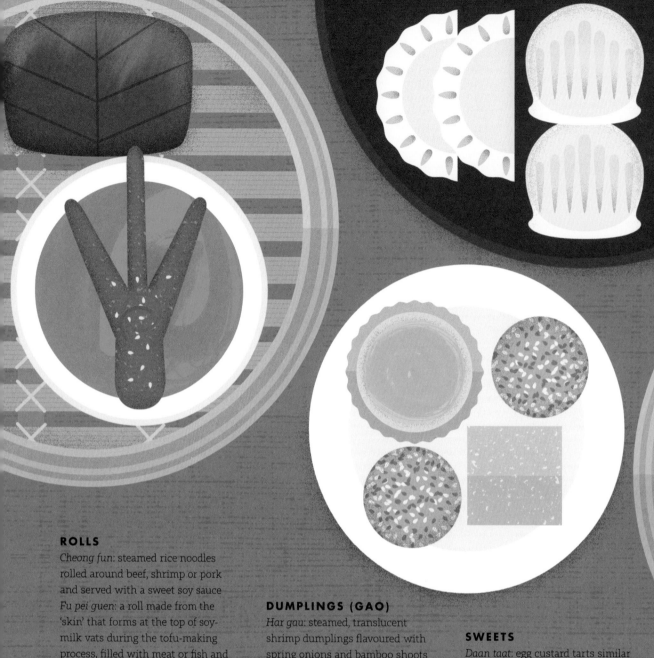

ROLLS

Cheong fun: steamed rice noodles rolled around beef, shrimp or pork and served with a sweet soy sauce

Fu pei guen: a roll made from the 'skin' that forms at the top of soy-milk vats during the tofu-making process, filled with meat or fish and either steamed or deep-fried

Lo mai gai: steamed glutinous rice mixed with spring onions, chicken, mushrooms and Chinese sausage, served on a lotus or banana leaf

Fung zao: fried and steamed chicken feet known as 'phoenix talons', served in a sweet and sour black bean or soy bean sauce

Pai gwut: tiny pieces of pork rib, steamed with fermented soy beans until they achieve a moist, slippery texture. Beware of the bones!

DUMPLINGS (GAO)

Har gau: steamed, translucent shrimp dumplings flavoured with spring onions and bamboo shoots

Chiu chow fun guo: crunchy, steamed dumplings filled with pork, shrimp and peanuts, and flavoured with coriander and jicama (Mexican turnip)

Siu mai: open-topped steamed pork or shrimp dumplings often garnished with carrot or fish roe

Ham sui gok: deep-fried rice and pork dumplings

Wu gok: crispy, semi-sweet fried taro dumplings with a savoury pork filling

SWEETS

Daan taat: egg custard tarts similar to Portuguese ones but more assertive and eggier in flavour

Jin deui: fried, rice-flour pastry balls, virtually identical to Japanese mochi. Filled with a sweet lotus or red bean paste

Dau fu fa: a soft pudding made from silken tofu, flavoured with a ginger or plain sugar syrup

Ma lai go: steamed sponge cake originally from Malaysia

Lai wong bao: steamed and filled custard buns

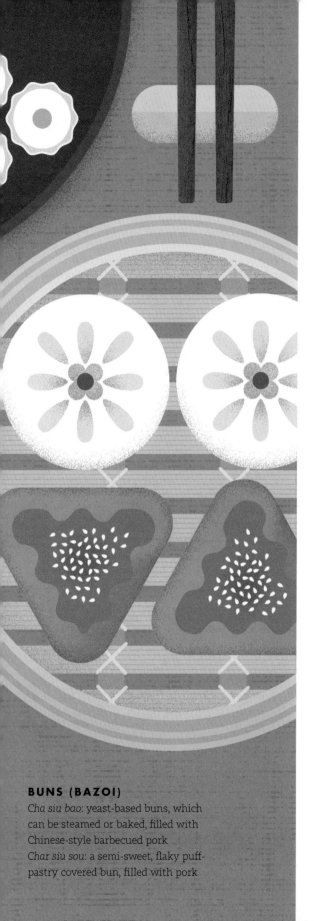

DIM SUM: DIP WHILE YOU SIP

The perfect pick-me-up, dim sum was originally created by the Cantonese to restore field workers and weary travellers with road-side eateries opening up as early as 5am to serve tea alongside a pick 'n' mix of sweet and savoury snacks. Traditionally a breakfast or brunch food, these days, and especially in the West, it is just as likely to be lunchtime tourists or savvy professionals between meetings, selecting from the rolling trolleys that the wide variety of dim sum are served from.

Whichever camp you might fall into, dim sum should ideally be enjoyed in numbers, with each small dish featuring just three or four bitesize pieces, making them perfect for sharing tapas-style. Order lots and across the menu, being sure not to bloat on the accompanying sticky rice-laden leaves. (Think of it as the bread basket of the East). And forget convention when it comes to the order of business: here savoury and sweet sit happily side by side.

DIP ON

Perhaps the best bit about dim sum, though, is the dipping: choose from spicy, sweet or salty

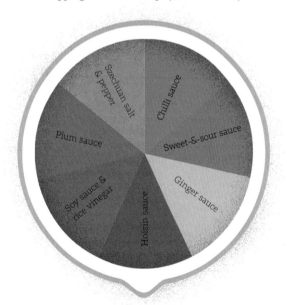

TEA TIME

The words 'dim' and 'sum' might literally mean 'point to your heart' but eating dim sum is also known as 'yum cha' in Cantonese or 'drink tea', and when you visit a dim sum restaurant you will always be offered a choice of char to sip with your meal

BUNS (BAZOI)

Cha siu bao: yeast-based buns, which can be steamed or baked, filled with Chinese-style barbecued pork
Char siu sou: a semi-sweet, flaky puff-pastry covered bun, filled with pork

—

SANDWICH: FINGER FOOD

The fourth Earl of Sandwich, notorious gambler, wanted a portable, handheld snack and it was this seemingly simple invention (most probably inspired by the people of the Mediterranean who had been nibbling mezze with flatbread for centuries) that has become a perennial favourite. Indeed, so convenient was this new finger food that it now continues to be one of the most popular 'fast foods' around the world. Believe it or not, sandwich shop chain Subway has more branches globally than McDonald's.

But for a sandwich to be really successful we need to return to its architecture. Whether we're talking cookies and ice cream, or the softest bao bun filled with sticky pork belly, it's important to construct your sandwich correctly. Layer your fillings incorrectly or be overzealous with your mayo and that heavenly slice can turn into a soggy mess.

BUILD-A-BUTTY

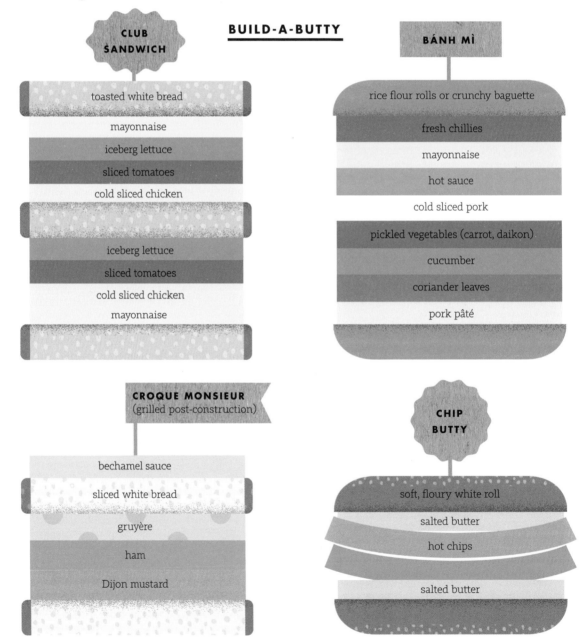

CLUB SANDWICH

- toasted white bread
- mayonnaise
- iceberg lettuce
- sliced tomatoes
- cold sliced chicken
- iceberg lettuce
- sliced tomatoes
- cold sliced chicken
- mayonnaise

BÁNH MÌ

- rice flour rolls or crunchy baguette
- fresh chillies
- mayonnaise
- hot sauce
- cold sliced pork
- pickled vegetables (carrot, daikon)
- cucumber
- coriander leaves
- pork pâté

CROQUE MONSIEUR
(grilled post-construction)

- bechamel sauce
- sliced white bread
- gruyère
- ham
- Dijon mustard

CHIP BUTTY

- soft, floury white roll
- salted butter
- hot chips
- salted butter

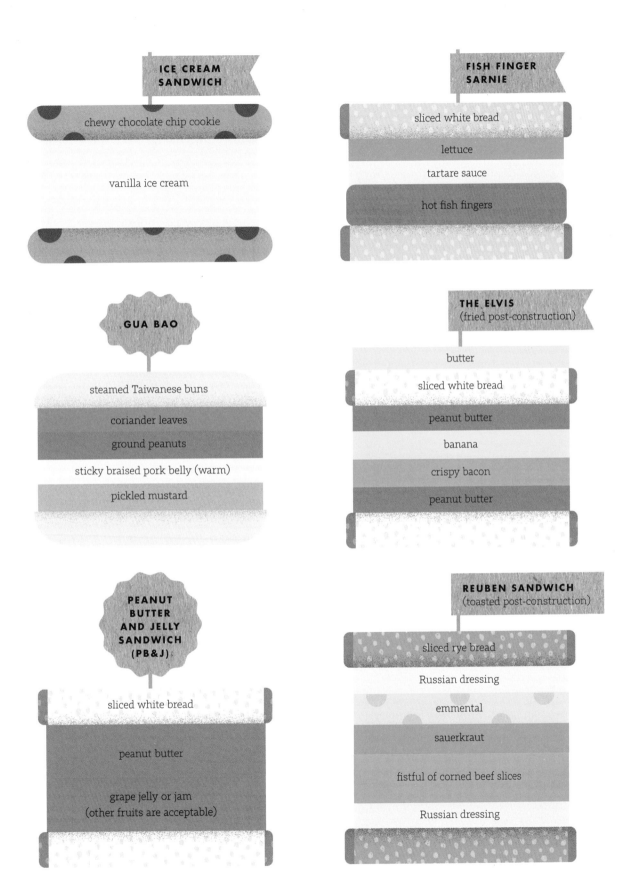

ICE CREAM SANDWICH

chewy chocolate chip cookie

vanilla ice cream

FISH FINGER SARNIE

sliced white bread

lettuce

tartare sauce

hot fish fingers

GUA BAO

steamed Taiwanese buns

coriander leaves

ground peanuts

sticky braised pork belly (warm)

pickled mustard

THE ELVIS
(fried post-construction)

butter

sliced white bread

peanut butter

banana

crispy bacon

peanut butter

PEANUT BUTTER AND JELLY SANDWICH (PB&J)

sliced white bread

peanut butter

grape jelly or jam
(other fruits are acceptable)

REUBEN SANDWICH
(toasted post-construction)

sliced rye bread

Russian dressing

emmental

sauerkraut

fistful of corned beef slices

Russian dressing

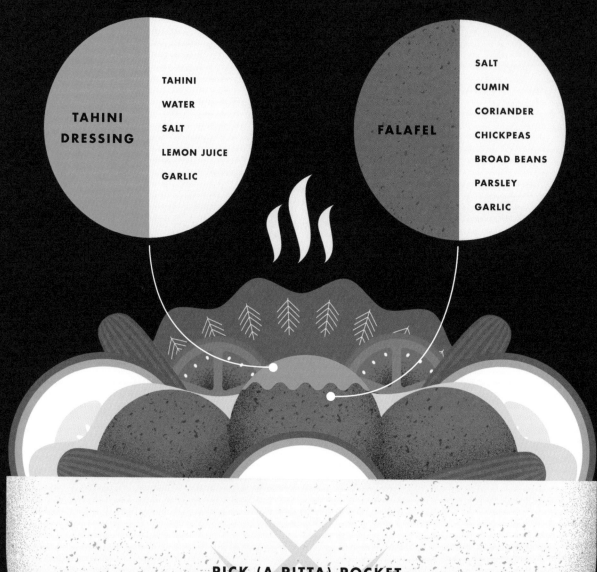

TAHINI DRESSING

- TAHINI
- WATER
- SALT
- LEMON JUICE
- GARLIC

FALAFEL

- SALT
- CUMIN
- CORIANDER
- CHICKPEAS
- BROAD BEANS
- PARSLEY
- GARLIC

PICK (A PITTA) POCKET

Fill your pitta pocket with a smear of hummus
(see page 138), sliced tomatoes, crunchy
cucumber, crisp Iceberg lettuce, hot falafels and
a drizzle of tahini sauce. Like it spicy? Add a hot
sauce, like Israel's green-chilli-based zhoug

—

FALAFEL: DITCH THE MEAT

For anyone that thinks vegan food is all about boring raw carrot sticks, point them in the direction of a hot, fried falafel stuffed into the pocket of a toasted flatbread with creamy hummus, salad and pickles. There's nothing virtuous about this Middle Eastern street food.

Originally from Egypt, where they are called ta'amia, the authentic falafel had nothing to do with chickpeas at all. The falafel was made using dried, skinned broad beans only, which kept them soft and together. It was the rest of the Levant that introduced chickpeas for their nutty flavour and texture – either using a combination of the pulses or swapping them completely – and Israel has adopted the latter as something of a national dish.

While even ancient falafel recipes vary from state to state, home to home, modern interpretations break tradition altogether. Today chefs and home cooks alike combine all manner of vegetables with chickpeas in this most simple of pastes – from sweet potato and squash to beetroot, red peppers or spinach, some even adding cheese.

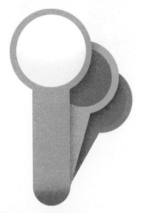

KEEP IT LIGHT

A raising agent like bicarbonate of soda or baking powder will help keep your falafels light and fluffy

HOLD IT TOGETHER

Tinned chickpeas have no place in falafels – they need to be uncooked, dried and then soaked overnight before pulsing until smooth. A little bit of roughness isn't a problem though, that'll just give your patty extra texture

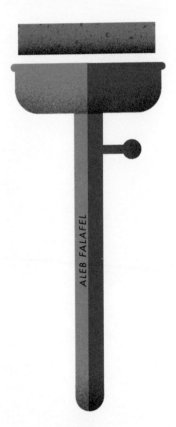

ALEB FALAFEL

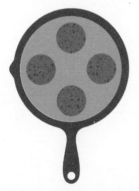

FRY OR NOT TO FRY?

You might spot recipes for shallow-fried or baked falafels but these are healthy imposters. Stick to deep-frying at 180°C in vegetable oil, before draining on kitchen towel

REST UP

Let the falafel mix rest before and after moulding for the best results

SHAPE SHIFTER

Moulding your falafels into the perfect shape is important if you want them cooked all the way through. Traditionally an 'aleb falafel' is used, otherwise you can create quenelles between two spoons, or roll your mix into flattened golf-ball-size patties

THE RAMEN RULES

In every ramen there are the same key components to achieve that perfect umami harmony of salty, fatty, carbtastic, deliciousness

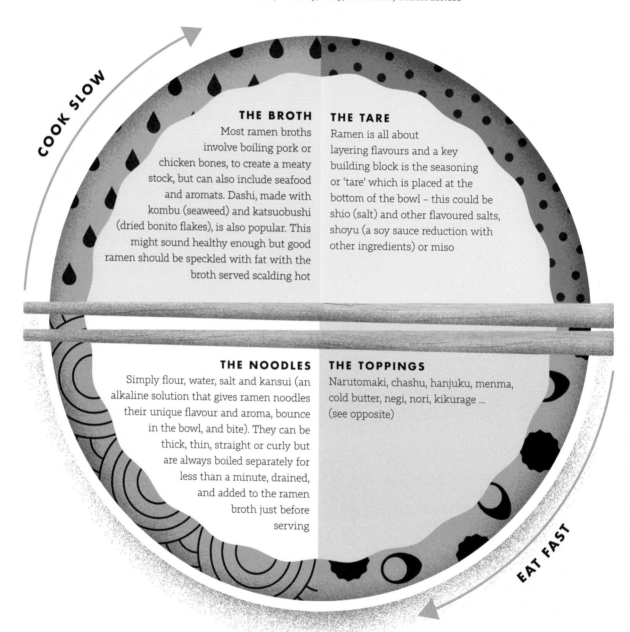

COOK SLOW

THE BROTH

Most ramen broths involve boiling pork or chicken bones, to create a meaty stock, but can also include seafood and aromats. Dashi, made with kombu (seaweed) and katsuobushi (dried bonito flakes), is also popular. This might sound healthy enough but good ramen should be speckled with fat with the broth served scalding hot

THE TARE

Ramen is all about layering flavours and a key building block is the seasoning or 'tare' which is placed at the bottom of the bowl – this could be shio (salt) and other flavoured salts, shoyu (a soy sauce reduction with other ingredients) or miso

THE NOODLES

Simply flour, water, salt and kansui (an alkaline solution that gives ramen noodles their unique flavour and aroma, bounce in the bowl, and bite). They can be thick, thin, straight or curly but are always boiled separately for less than a minute, drained, and added to the ramen broth just before serving

THE TOPPINGS

Narutomaki, chashu, hanjuku, menma, cold butter, negi, nori, kikurage … (see opposite)

EAT FAST

KNOW YOUR RAMEN:

There are around 30 different regional varieties of ramen in Japan alone (the most famous being Tokyo ramen) so make sure you start by learning the four basic types of ramen to order

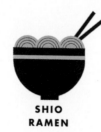

SHIO RAMEN

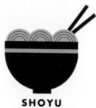

SHOYU RAMEN

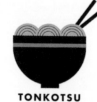

TONKOTSU RAMEN

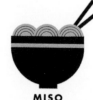

MISO RAMEN

RAMEN TOPPINGS

Narutomaki
Fish cake

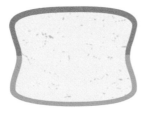

Chashu
Sliced pork belly

Hanjuku
Very soft boiled egg

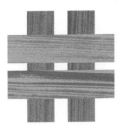

Menma
Cured bamboo shoots

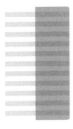

Cold butter

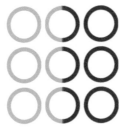

Negi
Shredded spring onions

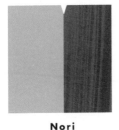

Nori
Dark seaweed sheets

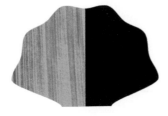

Kikurage
Black wood-ear mushroom

BONE BROTH FACIAL

There's no messing about with ramen. You must slurp and you must splatter with speed. Wait too long and those perfectly cooked noodles will go soft and flabby. Regular ramen eaters will have a burnt roof of their mouth and sweat on their brow from their steaming bone broth facial

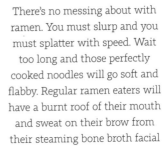

ON THE TABLE

—

RAMEN: ROCK AND ROLL NOODLES

Fans of the instant stuff might think that ramen is just noodle soup. But, go fresh and you'll never look back. This is cook-slow, eat-fast food. Broths can be boiled for up to 20 hours, rounds of dough can be hand-pulled into the thinnest noodles, egg yolks can be so softly boiled that their golden yolks are almost as smooth as custard, and pork belly so gently cooked (simply for the final flourish of garnish) that its sweet, melting fat will give you a deliciously greasy smile.

Such is its popularity, in fact, that there are thought to be more than 34,000 ramen shops across Japan alone (4,000 of which are in Tokyo). Not bad for some noodles that were brought to the country little over a century ago with the Chinese. Now, 100-odd years later, and the Japanese have claimed the dish as their own, with regional variants evolving all over the country. There's even a ramen museum in Shin-Yokohama. It's gone global too and mutated far beyond the bowl – there's been a ramen burger, a ramen pizza, taco, burrito and even a pudding.

But what does real ramen look and taste like? Just follow our ramen rules. And then break them: that's much more fun.

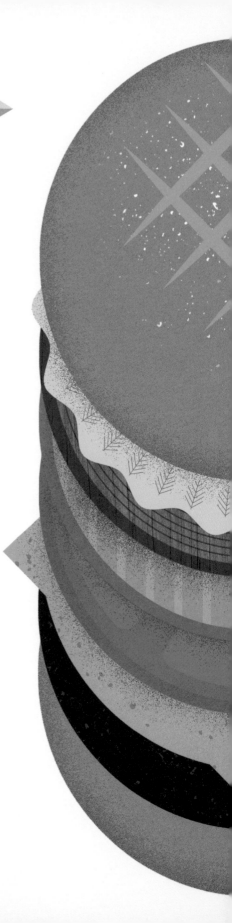

BURGERS: THE ORIGINAL FAST FOOD

There can be few foods around the world that are so significant that they inspire international franchises, TV shows, science experiments and global economy indexes; but, then again, there are few foods as deeply satisfying as a good burger.

In the last decade the humble burger – essentially, glorified beef and bread – has had something of a renaissance. It's gone gourmet, dirty (in a good way). No longer is any ol' bit of cow acceptable: the fat to meat ratio is crucial. The bun needs to be as good as the meat, and then there's the fillings – what about the cheese, bacon, pickles and salad? Chefs started getting creative, adding more meat to the stack – pulled pork, chilli con carne, foie gras and even lobster. Sauces made the leap from mustard and ketchup to truffled mayonnaise. Gherkins morphed into Korean kimchi. It all got rather complicated. But what actually makes the perfect burger? Here's our guide…

THE ANTIPODEAN BURGER:
Make like the Australians do and fill your stack with pickled beetroot, sliced pineapple, a fried egg and chilli. Really

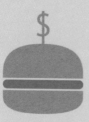

BURGERNOMICS:
The Big Mac Index has been used since 1986 by *The Economist* to show global purchasing power

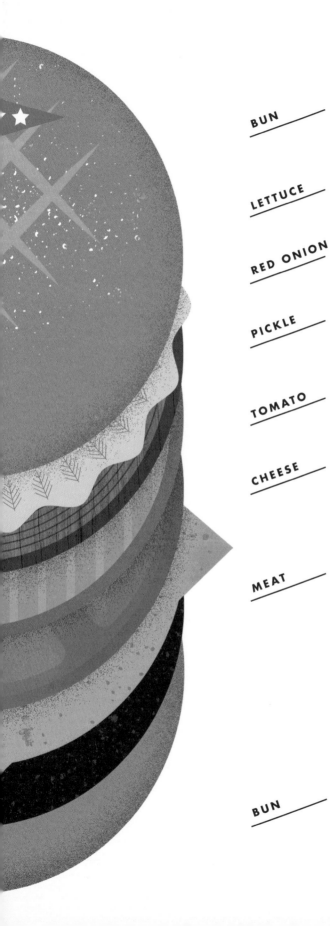

BUN — The perfect bap for a burger needs to be strong enough to hold its generous filling and should be slightly sweet. Look out for rolls with a hint of sourdough. Toast on the same pan/grill as your patty

LETTUCE — Keep it green and crisp. Add the freshest leaves of iceberg lettuce, straight from the fridge, at the last minute to ensure no wilting

RED ONION — Sliced thinly, and quickly pickled in red wine vinegar and caster sugar, red onion hum will make your burger sing

PICKLE — You need something sharp to cut through all that delicious meat. Try crinkle-cut pickled gherkins (good for texture and sourness) or a homemade cucumber pickle

TOMATO — Beef, plum or roma, whatever the variety of tomato, they must be ripe and sliced around 5mm at room temperature with a serrated knife

CHEESE — Even the top chefs can't resist the melt of 'plastic' sliced cheese but for the same consistency with extra flavour choose a Gouda. Slice thin, larger than the size of your burger and be sure to add to the top of the cooked patty the second it is flipped over. In the time it takes to cook the other side you'll have the perfect melt

MEAT — Beef. Always. Make it chuck steak (the shoulder of the cow) and you'll have the perfect meat to fat ratio (around 20–25% fat). Coarsely hand grind it, or ask your butcher to do it for you. Add just salt and pepper: no egg, breadcrumbs, beer, herbs or spices. Mix to combine but don't overwork it. Shape into rough 250g patties (that's a handful or ice-cream scoop) and make a dimple in the middle. Cover and chill for 30 minutes – burgers should always be cooked from cold. A skillet or barbecue grill should be your weapon of choice, over a hot heat. Cook for 2–3 minutes on the first side – don't be tempted to move it or press down on the meat – and then flip it for a final 1 minute on the other side

BUN — Don't forget the burger to bun ratio! Lockjaw burgers are all well and good on paper but a sloppy mess in reality. A burger should always be a cutlery free affair

SALAD: BECOME A BUILDER

Learn how to layer when it comes to crafting the perfect salad.

THE BUILDING BLOCKS: VEG TO BREAD

Don't let the same old ingredients languish at the bottom of your salad drawer. Mix your salads up with proteins, fruit and veg, crunchy nuts and seeds and croutons. The perfect salad demands a rich variety of colour, texture and flavours

THE CEMENT: VINAIGRETTE

A good dressing will bring together all of your salad building blocks. Dress sturdy cabbages and kales 1-2 hours before serving; coat cooked salad items like sliced new potatoes while still warm; but dress delicate leaves at the very last minute to avoid wilting and a soggy end salad

THE FOUNDATIONS: GREENS

The base of any salad (its leafy greens, whether delicate herbs, hardy kales, or crisp lettuce) will dictate the direction of the final dish. Pick radicchio and you'll need to balance the bitter, opt for citrusy sorrel and you might like to counteract with something creamy, while peppery rocket can share plate space with very flavourful additions. Treat delicate leaves and herbs with care; while cabbages and kales can be finely shredded raw or lightly blanched and served warm

THE PROTEIN

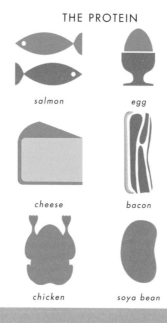

salmon · egg · cheese · bacon · chicken · soya bean

THE VEG

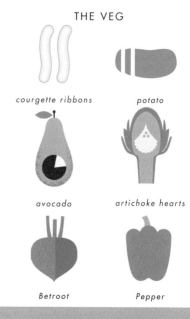

courgette ribbons · potato · avocado · artichoke hearts · Betroot · Pepper

THE ALL ROUNDER

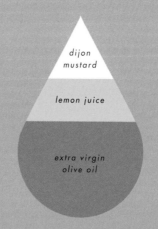

dijon mustard
lemon juice
extra virgin olive oil

THE SWEET TALKER

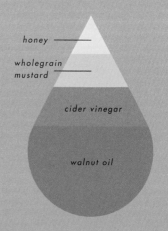

honey
wholegrain mustard
cider vinegar
walnut oil

IF YOU LIKE IT PEPPERY

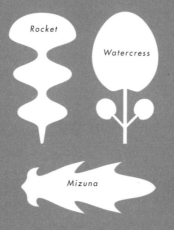

Rocket · Watercress · Mizuna

IF YOU CRAVE TEXTURE

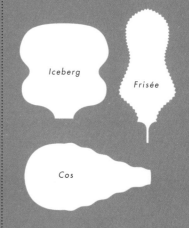

Iceberg · Frisée · Cos

THE FRUIT

nectarine

orange/
pink grapefruit

pear

watermelon

apple

Pomegranite seeds

THE CRUNCH

croutons

pitta shards

walnuts

roasted chickpeas

pine nut

pumpkin seeds

THE FINAL FLOURISH

mint

basil

coriander

dill

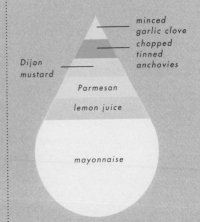
edible flowers

chives

THE GLOBETROTTER

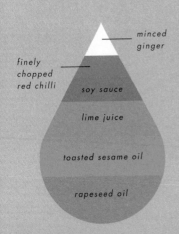

minced ginger

finely chopped red chilli

soy sauce

lime juice

toasted sesame oil

rapeseed oil

THE RANCHER

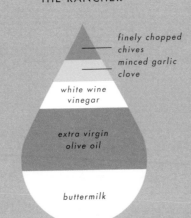

finely chopped chives

minced garlic clove

white wine vinegar

extra virgin olive oil

buttermilk

THE SIMPLE CAESAR

minced garlic clove

chopped tinned anchovies

Dijon mustard

Parmesan

lemon juice

mayonnaise

IF YOU'RE BITTER

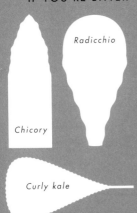

Radicchio

Chicory

Curly kale

IF YOU WANT IT SIMPLE

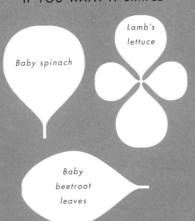

Lamb's lettuce

Baby spinach

Baby beetroot leaves

THE WILD CARDS

White & red cabbage

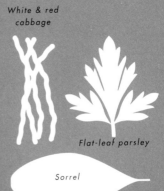

Flat-leaf parsley

Sorrel

PIZZA: THE WORLD IS FLAT AND ROUND

While the home of good pizza nowadays might be thought of as Naples – order a marinara rather than a Margherita for a truly authentic taste (tomatoes, oregano, garlic and extra virgin olive oil) – people across the Med have been eating flatbreads topped with ingredients since the classical period. And, after the Italians nailed the recipe, it's travelled ever since.

The secret to a perfect pizza, though, whatever interpretation you might take, is a piping hot oven. Professionals prefer wood-fired, which can get up to temperatures of 400°C but if you're at home, just crank the oven up as hot as it will go. To ensure a crispy base, preheat a pizza stone, metal griddle or thick flat oven tray, and don't overload your pizza with toppings or it won't cook through evenly.

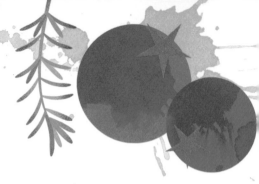

BUILD YOUR BASE

The Graceland of pizza might be in the Italian port of Naples but there's more to this flatbread than the tricolore Margherita. Why not take inspiration from around the world?

Start with basic pizza dough + tomato and garlic sauce + ...

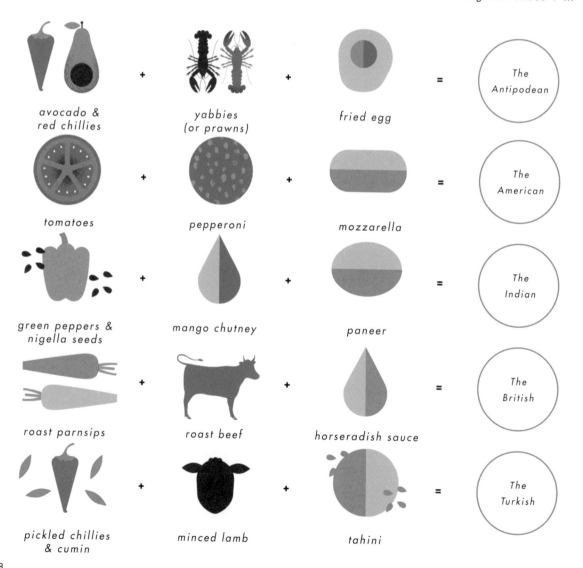

avocado & red chillies +	yabbies (or prawns) +	fried egg =	The Antipodean
tomatoes +	pepperoni +	mozzarella =	The American
green peppers & nigella seeds +	mango chutney +	paneer =	The Indian
roast parsnips +	roast beef +	horseradish sauce =	The British
pickled chillies & cumin +	minced lamb +	tahini =	The Turkish

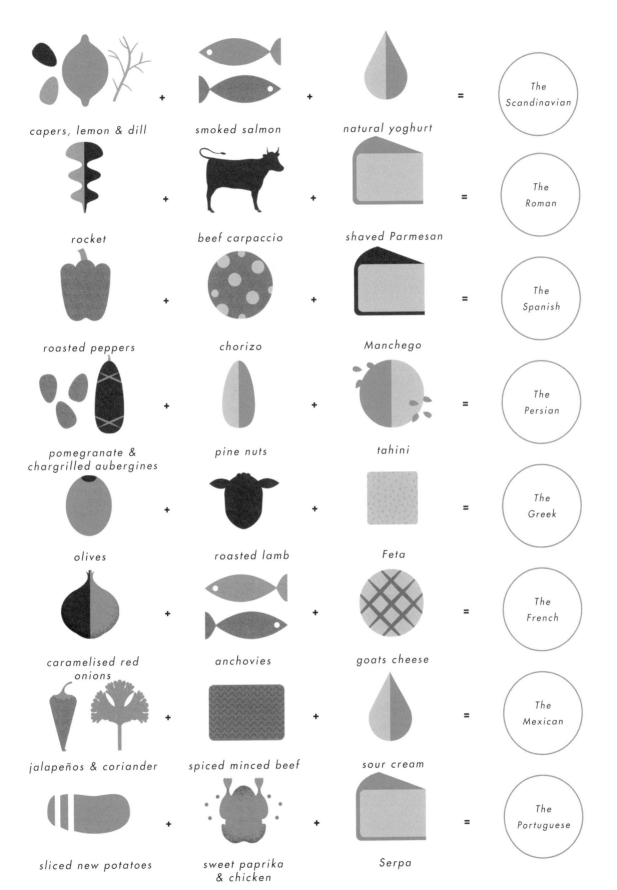

capers, lemon & dill + smoked salmon + natural yoghurt = The Scandinavian

rocket + beef carpaccio + shaved Parmesan = The Roman

roasted peppers + chorizo + Manchego = The Spanish

pomegranate & chargrilled aubergines + pine nuts + tahini = The Persian

olives + roasted lamb + Feta = The Greek

caramelised red onions + anchovies + goats cheese = The French

jalapeños & coriander + spiced minced beef + sour cream = The Mexican

sliced new potatoes + sweet paprika & chicken + Serpa = The Portuguese

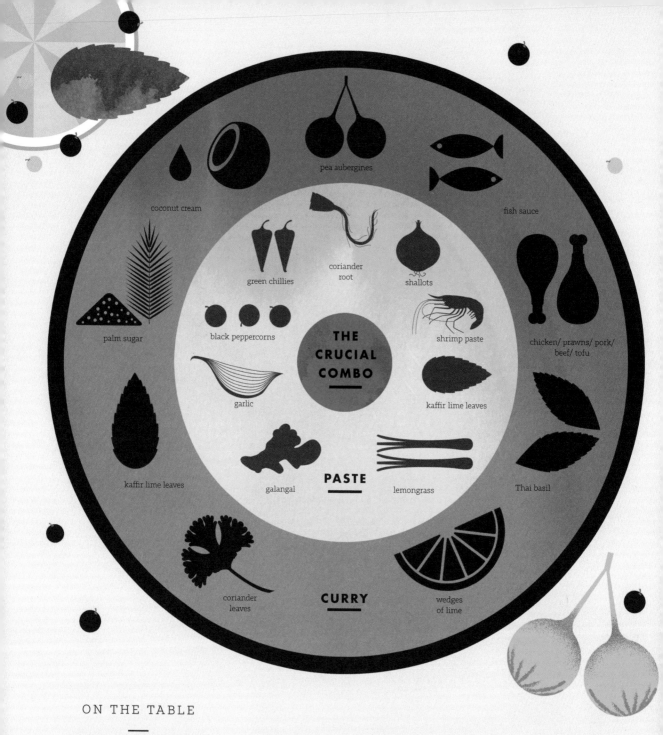

pea aubergines

fish sauce

coconut cream

green chillies

coriander root

shallots

palm sugar

black peppercorns

shrimp paste

chicken/ prawns/ pork/ beef/ tofu

THE CRUCIAL COMBO

garlic

kaffir lime leaves

kaffir lime leaves

galangal

PASTE

lemongrass

Thai basil

coriander leaves

CURRY

wedges of lime

ON THE TABLE

GREEN THAI CURRY: SPICING THINGS UP

Thai green curry is bold, fiery, sweet, sour, salty and comforting all at the same time, and unlike its culinary cousins elsewhere in Asia, luxuriates in liquid. The secret to a perfect Thai green curry changes depending on the household you're speaking to but the starting point is always the paste. It's easy to make your own from scratch nowadays, with all of the essential ingredients (from aromatic kaffir lime leaves and lemongrass to sweet palm sugar and umami-rich fish sauce) now widely available in supermarkets and online. The protein or bulk of the curry can be whatever you like – from king prawns to tofu cubes or a handful of seasonal veg – but if you're sticking to tradition make sure everything is bitesize. This is a dish to be eaten with a fork and spoon.

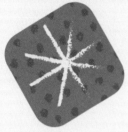

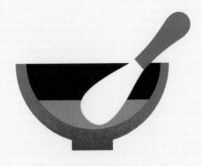

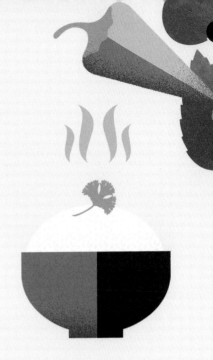

FIRE AND ICE

If you're going to the trouble of making Thai green curry paste from scratch, be sure to make extra. Store in the fridge, in a sterilized jar, with a layer of flavourless oil covering the paste, or spoon into an ice cube tray and freeze for later

POUND FOR POUND

There's a time and a place for modern convenience and this paste isn't one of them. If you want a shortcut buy a readymade one, but if you truly want to make it from scratch you need to pound each ingredient together using a pestle and mortar. No food processors allowed. The former teases out each component's essential oils and combines them into a fragrant, homogenous explosion of flavours; while a chopper will simply chop

RICE, RICE BABY

Rice plays an important part in Thai cuisine and can be served sticky or steamed. Look for jasmine rice in the supermarkets

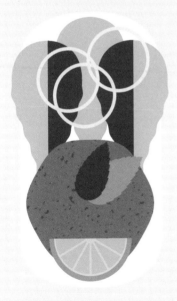

BEST OF THE REST

Like green curry? You'll love these other great Thai dishes

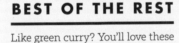

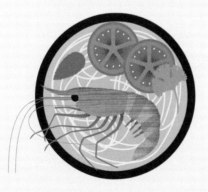

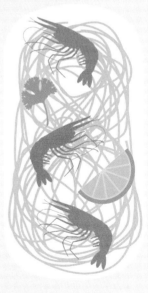

LARB

A crispy, spicy warm salad of minced meat (pork, beef, chicken or turkey) served on crisp lettuce leaves

TOM YUM

An aromatic, searingly spicy and sour soup flavoured with lemongrass, lime and chillies – a sure-fire way to clear the sinuses

PAD THAI

Fried noodles with garlic, fish sauce, eggs, dried shrimps, beansprouts, roasted peanuts and whatever protein takes your fancy (prawns and pork work well)

PASTIES: HANDHELD EAT

Some foods were made to be enjoyed on fine crockery, others were designed to be scoffed on the hoof, hand to pie hole, as adventure fuel. And what better fast food is there than buttery pastry stuffed with a hot, deeply savoury filling?

The first pasties appeared in England in the 13th century; traditionally a hardy shortcrust pastry filled with vegetables (meat was too expensive) and later anything from chicken and venison to eel and even (honestly) porpoise.

Its most famous incarnation though is the Cornish pasty. Distinctively D-shaped, crimped around the edges and packed with (if we're being authentic) chunks of beef, swede, potato, onion and plenty of black pepper – it's a dish that's been quoted in English literature, Shakespeare no less, and translated around the world. So special is it, that it's even been awarded a protected food name status alongside Scottish salmon, Champagne and Stilton cheese.

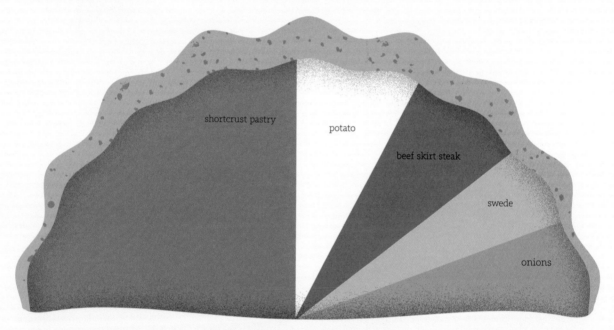

ENGLAND – CORNISH PASTY

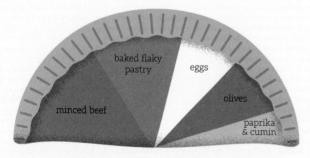

ARGENTINA – EMPANADA

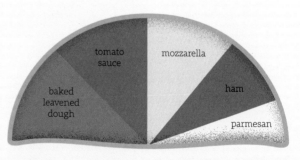

ITALY – CALZONE

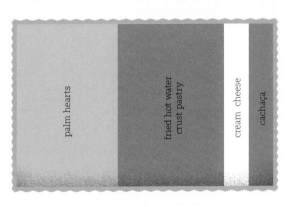

BRAZIL – PASTEL

palm hearts | fried hot water crust pastry | cream cheese | cachaça

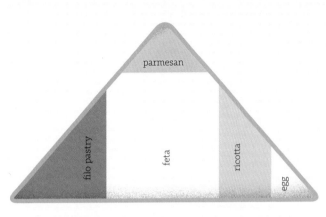

GREECE – TYROPITÁKIA

parmesan | filo pastry | feta | ricotta | egg

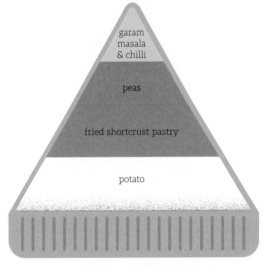

INDIA – SAMOSA

garam masala & chilli | peas | fried shortcrust pastry | potato

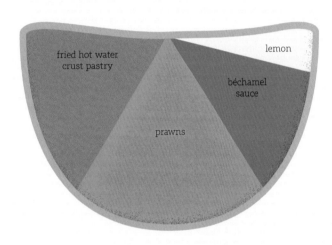

PORTUGAL – RISSOLE

fried hot water crust pastry | lemon | béchamel sauce | prawns

TURKEY – BÖREK

filo | feta | parsley

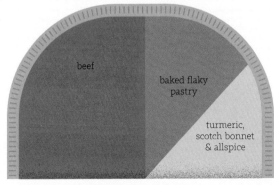

JAMAICA – PATTY

beef | baked flaky pastry | turmeric, scotch bonnet & allspice

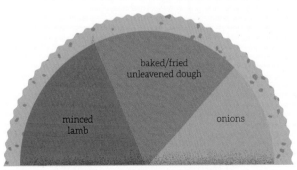

RUSSIA – CHIBUREKKI

baked/fried unleavened dough | minced lamb | onions

—

SUSHI: ROLL WITH IT

Perfect sushi starts with perfect rice – short grain Japanese rice, boiled and steamed until tender and sticky, and seasoned with salt, sugar and rice vinegar. It is then rolled, topped or moulded with raw and/or cooked fish and shellfish, vegetables, pickles, and (more recently in the West) meat, too. It can be encased in nori (sheets of dried seaweed) and decorated with any number of garnishes – from bright orange fish roe to black sesame seeds and mayonnaise.

Traditionally wasabi paste (a root with a fiery burn) is incorporated into the sushi but can also be served on the side, along with soy sauce and pickled ginger, which was originally meant to be a palate cleanser between each type of sushi. Japanese chefs train for a minimum of two years to master the techniques needed to create the perfect rolls and etiquette dictates a correct way of eating it. But rules are made to be broken... Except for the one that says dip your nigiri fish-side into the soy sauce – only a fool will ignore that advice, and be left with collapsed rice and an embarrassed grin.

MAKE YOUR OWN: YOU WILL NEED

Damp fingers make easy work of sticky sushi rice

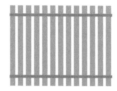

Roll tightly in a bamboo mat and slice to order to keep it fresh

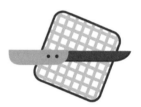

Make clean cuts with a sharp, wet knife – wipe clean after every slice

KEY

FISH/SEAFOOD

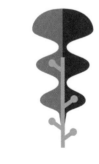

NORI

SUSHI RICE

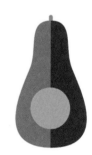

VEGETABLES

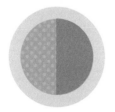

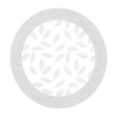

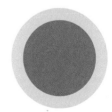

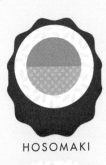

HOSOMAKI

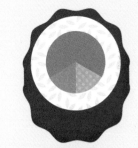

MAKI

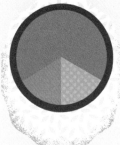

URAMAKI

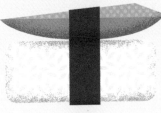

NIGIRI

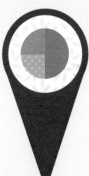

TEMAKI

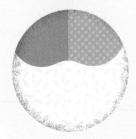

TEMARI

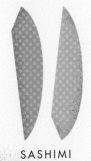

SASHIMI

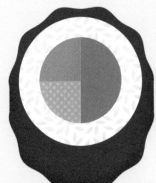

FUTOMAKI

STEW: A MELTING POT

This dish is all about long, slow cooking, allowing the stars of the show (often meat, and sometimes vegetables) to become tender, and the various spices, herbs and aromatics to amalgamate into a rich and wholesome sauce. It's a taste of home, a staple of winter and a surprisingly cheap and easy way to cook.

1. THE MAIN EVENT

For friends of fish
Choose a variety of sustainable fish (coley, mackerel and pollock) and shellfish (mussels and prawns) for a stew packed with flavour and texture. They need a short cook but a proper stock is essential

For vegetable lovers
Try aubergines and mushrooms, alongside lentils, chickpeas and beans (haricot, cannellini and butter) for protein in the winter; peas, lettuce and courgette, with vibrant soft, fresh herbs (tarragon, chervil and chives) in the summer

For the carnivore
Beef shin, cheek, brisket and oxtail; lamb neck, breast, shoulder and shank; pork knuckle or shoulder; chicken thighs and legs; and whole rabbits and pheasants (who benefit from a liquid braise with their lean meat)

2. THE BACKBONE OF FLAVOUR

Herbs
Dry woody herbs such as bay, sage, rosemary and thyme should be added at the start and can be finely chopped or added whole, and removed at the end. Fish-loving fennel, dill or tarragon should be stirred through at the last minute

Holy trinity
Start any stew with onions, carrot and celery and you can't go far wrong. Garlic is also great for adding mellow round-edness

Booze
Pork and rabbit like cider or dry sherry with a mustard and cream sauce, beef is keen on red wine or ale and fish or game birds work well with a slog of vermouth

Salty kick
Seasoning is a must but you can add some real savoury flavour with a small amount of cured meats – think bacon, pancetta, guanciale, Italian sausages, chorizo

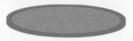

3. THE BODY

Grains

Pearl barley, farro and freekeh or tiny pastas like orzo don't just add body; they also give great texture to stew. Experiment with tiny pseudo-grains like quinoa, buckwheat or amaranth for a lighter version of the traditional stew

Pulses

Beans and lentils add protein, are a cheap way to bulk out the stew, and keep you fuller for longer

Potatoes

They're cheap, filling and they also absorb the flavours around them; choose whole new potatoes to avoid them completely disintegrating

Dumplings

Whether made from suet, flour and water, or more adventurous ingredients like saffron, semolina and Parmesan, these are a rib-sticking crowning glory to any stew. Add herbs, citrus zest and spices to taste

Vegetables

Small pearl onions, chunks of root vegetables like parsnips, sweet potato, squash or turnip add variety to winter stews

4. THE COOKING

1. Kickstart the Maillard reaction by browning meat over a high heat. Caramelisation pumps up the flavour but after that the rule of thumb is low and slow. Try roasting vegetables prior to placing in the casserole dish – just add them at the end of cooking so that they retain their shape

2. The liquid should be just trembling in the centre of the pot, over the hob or in the oven. Better yet, try a slow cooker, which is great for low-energy cooking

3. Add ingredients according to their cooking time – meat and pre-soaked dried beans takes the longest, root vegetables and grains slightly less (ideally add them an hour before the end of cooking) and fresh vegetables like garden peas and pre-cooked beans near the end

5. TO FINISH

Keep it fresh: Try gremolata, persillade, a swirl of salsa verde, or chopped fresh soft herbs to add a fresh hit of flavour in your slow-cooked medley. Finely chopped preserved lemons can also add a delicious tang to summer fish

Up the flavour: Adding yoghurt, sour cream and crème fraîche upon serving can cut through any richness in stew. Try Greek yoghurt with a little crushed garlic, salt, herbs, lemon zest, olive oil and Tabasco

Cheese: Feta and goat's curd can make a vegetable stew sing, while hard cheeses are delicious grated on tomato-based or beery meat stews

PIE: THE IRRATIONAL DINNER

The fodder of choice for football matches and the subject of nursery rhymes, has another treat caused as much controversy as the pie? At once seemingly so simple – pastry encasing a sweet or savoury filling – it is yet so complex. It's neither folded, wrapped or free-standing (unless it's a pork pie) – a pie should be in a pie tin (either metal, to avoid a soggy bottom, or ceramic or china to avoid overbrowning), with pastry lining the top and bottom. Right? But what about modern pies, of essentially stews, served with a pastry 'top', or the key lime pie with no pastry at all? Whatever your predilection, perhaps just avoid one particular medieval tradition of pie making, where cooks were known to encase live birds as a surprise for their guests.

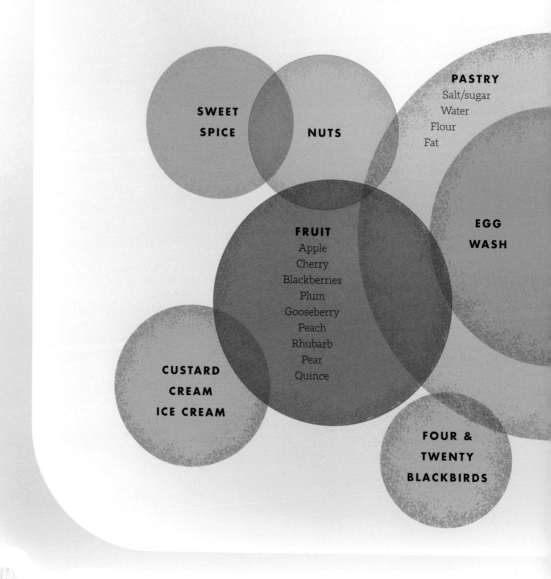

SWEET SPICE

NUTS

PASTRY
Salt/sugar
Water
Flour
Fat

FRUIT
Apple
Cherry
Blackberries
Plum
Gooseberry
Peach
Rhubarb
Pear
Quince

EGG WASH

CUSTARD CREAM ICE CREAM

FOUR & TWENTY BLACKBIRDS

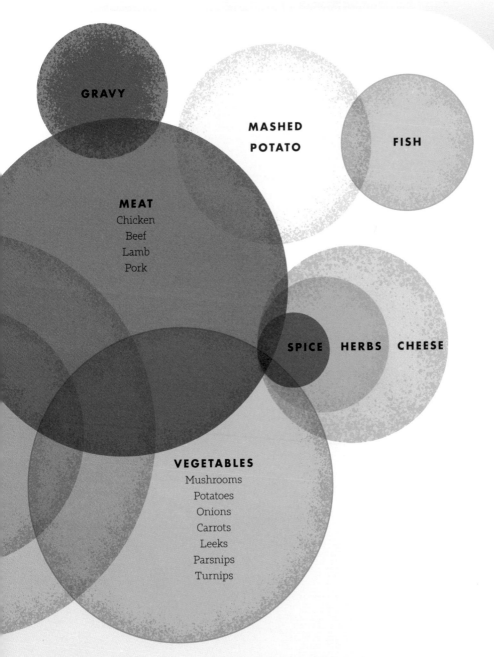

GRAVY

MASHED
POTATO

FISH

MEAT
Chicken
Beef
Lamb
Pork

SPICE   HERBS   CHEESE

VEGETABLES
Mushrooms
Potatoes
Onions
Carrots
Leeks
Parsnips
Turnips

- Blind baking the bottom layer of pastry can help avoid a soggy bottom
- Make savoury fillings in advance (ideally the day before) to allow the flavours to develop and the filling to cool before placing on the pastry base
- Crimping isn't just about making the pie look pretty but sealing in the filling too, so be firm
- Create a pie hole, either with a purpose-made pie funnel, or simply pierce the pastry top with a knife, to help steam escape and reduce spillages
- Brush sweet and savoury pie crusts with egg wash (egg beaten with milk) to create a shiny golden glaze

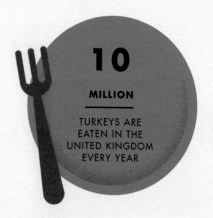

10

MILLION

TURKEYS ARE
EATEN IN THE
UNITED KINGDOM
EVERY YEAR

THERE IS A GENE
THAT DETERMINES
IF YOU WILL LOVE
OR HATE BRUSSELS
SPROUTS

TAS2R38

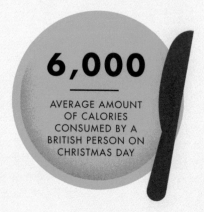

6,000

AVERAGE AMOUNT
OF CALORIES
CONSUMED BY A
BRITISH PERSON ON
CHRISTMAS DAY

ON THE TABLE

—

CHRISTMAS: A LUNCH OF EXCESS

In the Christian world there is one day in the calendar where families come together, regardless of age, gender or location, and feast. For some that means an informal barbecue on a beach, for others a ritualistic dinner linked to their faith. But for all there is a common theme – excess.

It can take months of planning and preparation. Christmas pudding, a tradition enjoyed in England since medieval times, begins its journey to the table on the last Sunday before Advent on 'Stir-up Sunday'. The cook is told to stir from east to west, in homage to the three wise men. Original recipes called for beef or mutton along with wine but most modern versions stick to a combination of dried fruits, spices and alcohol: 13 is the magic number, to represent Christ and the 12 Apostles. Some cooks add a silver coin to the mix to bring wealth and good luck upon the finder. And when it's finally served, up to 30 days later? Then it is decorated with holly, as a nod to Jesus's crown of thorns, and flamed with brandy to serve as the Passion.

Italy favours panforte, a sticky, spicy 'bread' dense with dried fruits, nuts and sugar from Siena, and panettone from Milan, a fluffy, fruity loaf cake.

Germany has a buttery, yeasted loaf with peel, spice, currants and marzipan called stollen, while in Greece you'll be offered melomakàrona. These lie somewhere between cakes and cookies, and are flavoured with olive oil, cinnamon and cloves, and drenched in nuts and honey.

For the majority of Christian countries around the world, though, the main event is decidedly savoury. Roast turkey is enduringly popular. In Britain it became a tradition sometime around the 1950s, when the bird became affordable and fridges commonplace. Before this time you were just as likely to find goose or beef as the centrepiece. In North America, it's served at Thanksgiving *and* Christmas, often with cranberry sauce; South America plate it with giblets and white rice; it's sliced cold in Australia; and roasted with various trimmings across most of Europe.

Other countries shun meat altogether for their celebrations. Italy has a feast of seven fishes on Christmas Eve, preferring salt cod, calamari and eel. In Lithuania, Poland, Ukraine and Belarus, they express their faith through 12 meatless dishes including pickled herrings, sour soup, freshwater fish, noodles and breads.

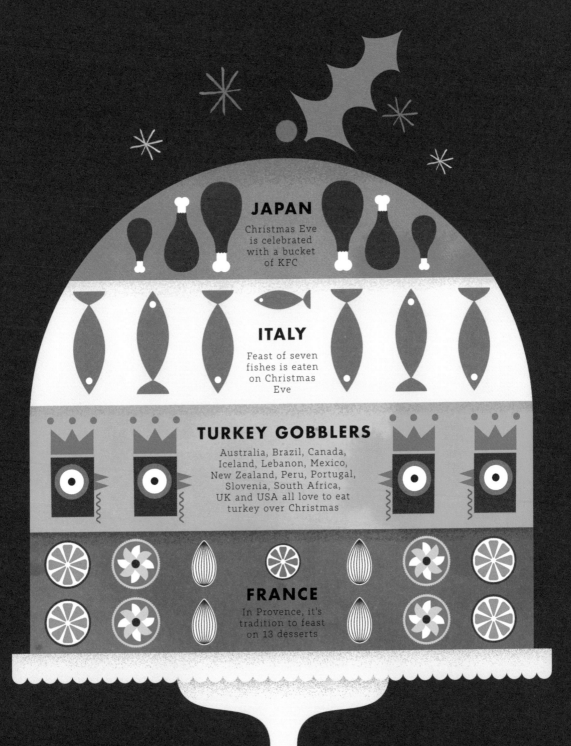

JAPAN
Christmas Eve is celebrated with a bucket of KFC

ITALY
Feast of seven fishes is eaten on Christmas Eve

TURKEY GOBBLERS
Australia, Brazil, Canada, Iceland, Lebanon, Mexico, New Zealand, Peru, Portugal, Slovenia, South Africa, UK and USA all love to eat turkey over Christmas

FRANCE
In Provence, it's tradition to feast on 13 desserts

FAT PANCAKES

Mix 135g plain flour with 1 egg, 130ml milk, 1 tsp baking powder, 2 tbsp caster sugar and 2 tbsp melted butter and whisk for a thicker batter. You want the consistency of thick double cream. Drop 1 heaped tbsp into a hot, buttered frying pan and fry for 1 minute until you begin to see bubbles on the surface. Flip or turn over and fry until golden brown and risen.

THE PERFECT MIX FOR THIN PANCAKES

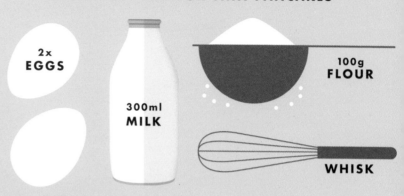

2x EGGS

300ml MILK

100g FLOUR

WHISK

FAT VS THIN: HOW DO YOU FRY YOURS?

SCOTCH PANCAKES

Also known as drop scones, these are small and traditionally cooked on a griddle or open hearth

BUTTERMILK PANCAKES

The USA and Canada's signature fat and fluffy pancake. Its secret weapon is baking powder, mixed with flour, buttermilk and sugar for a perfect puff

FAT

PANNENKOEKEN OR DUTCH BABY

A large family-sized sweet pancake from the Netherlands, baked soufflé-style in an oven. This pancake is egg heavy and needs to be served immediately before it collapses

AUSTRALIAN PIKELETS

Smaller than their Northern Hemisphere cousin, these thick pancakes are a popular snack down under, and are sometimes served afternoon-tea-style with jam and cream

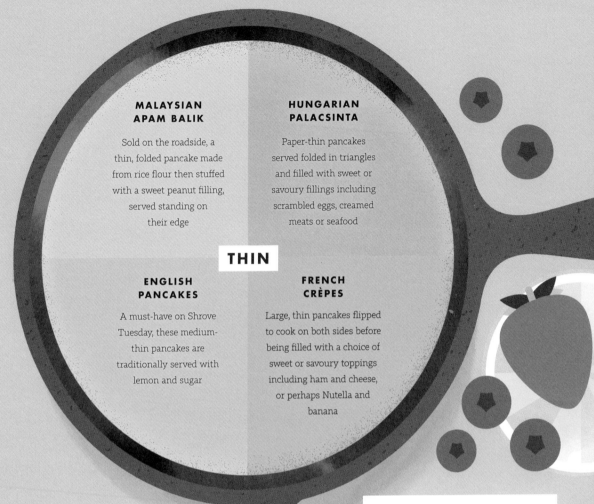

MALAYSIAN APAM BALIK

Sold on the roadside, a thin, folded pancake made from rice flour then stuffed with a sweet peanut filling, served standing on their edge

HUNGARIAN PALACSINTA

Paper-thin pancakes served folded in triangles and filled with sweet or savoury fillings including scrambled eggs, creamed meats or seafood

THIN

ENGLISH PANCAKES

A must-have on Shrove Tuesday, these medium-thin pancakes are traditionally served with lemon and sugar

FRENCH CRÊPES

Large, thin pancakes flipped to cook on both sides before being filled with a choice of sweet or savoury toppings including ham and cheese, or perhaps Nutella and banana

ON THE TABLE

PANCAKES: STACK 'EM HIGH

This original fast food is often associated with many religious festivals, including Shrove Tuesday and Hanukkah, with its few ingredients symbolizing big things: eggs for creation, flour the staff of life, salt wholesomeness and milk purity. It was also a celebratory way to use up the foods forbidden during Lent fasting.

Nowadays, of course, pancakes are a part of the everyday. Whether you like yours in the morning, fat, stacked high and covered in maple syrup like George Washington (reportedly). Or maybe you like yours mini, like bitesize buckwheat blinis topped with sour cream, smoked salmon and caviar. Or perhaps you're a fan of the thin, rolled and stuffed with shredded roast duck, hoisin sauce, cucumber, spring onions for dinner in a bao bing like the Chinese. There's a pancake for everyone and any time. But whichever way you like to eat yours, the question remains: do you flip high or slide low?

THIN PANCAKES

Mix 100g plain flour with 2 eggs, 300ml milk and 1 tbsp melted butter. Whisk thoroughly and rest for 30 minutes. You want the consistency of pouring single cream. When ready to cook, add a knob of unsalted butter to a non-stick frying pan. As it starts to melt, add a ladle of the rested batter and swirl the mix around the pan until it covers the entire base. Cook for 1-2 minutes before flipping, or gently turning over and repeat on the other side. Then bin it: the first pancake is always the worst. Repeat, and you'll have perfect pancakes for the rest of the batch. Serve with lemon juice and sugar or whatever takes your fancy.

MACARONS: MASTER THE MONSTER

Such simple creatures really; a blend of egg whites, sugar and almonds. Not to be confused with the macaroon, which despite its similar ingredients can be made in under 30 minutes, the macaron is an example of French patisserie at its most elegant and is best eaten some 52 hours after first cracking the eggs. There's very little room for error, but once you understand the principles behind each stage, you'll be making perfect macarons every time.

FILLING IDEAS

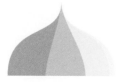

Lemon curd

Chocolate ganache

Flavoured buttercream

Fruit jam

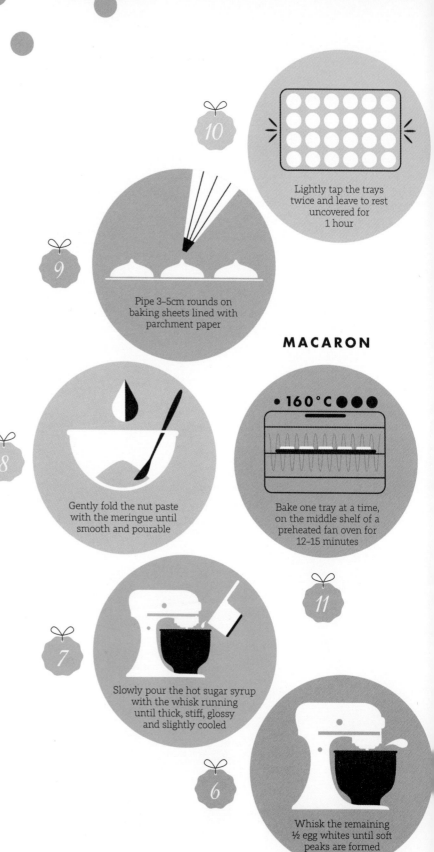

10 Lightly tap the trays twice and leave to rest uncovered for 1 hour

9 Pipe 3–5cm rounds on baking sheets lined with parchment paper

MACARON

8 Gently fold the nut paste with the meringue until smooth and pourable

160°C Bake one tray at a time, on the middle shelf of a preheated fan oven for 12-15 minutes

7 Slowly pour the hot sugar syrup with the whisk running until thick, stiff, glossy and slightly cooled

11

6 Whisk the remaining ½ egg whites until soft peaks are formed

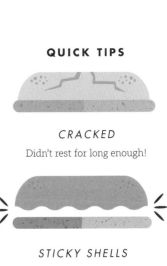

QUICK TIPS

CRACKED

Didn't rest for long enough!

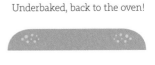

STICKY SHELLS

Underbaked, back to the oven!

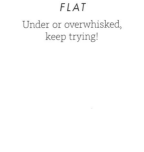

FLAT

Under or overwhisked,
keep trying!

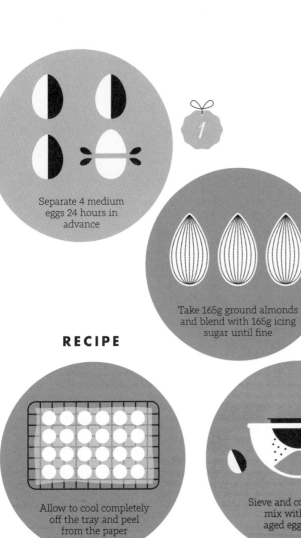

1

Separate 4 medium
eggs 24 hours in
advance

2

Take 165g ground almonds
and blend with 165g icing
sugar until fine

RECIPE

3

Sieve and combine the
mix with ½ the
aged egg whites

Allow to cool completely
off the tray and peel
from the paper

12

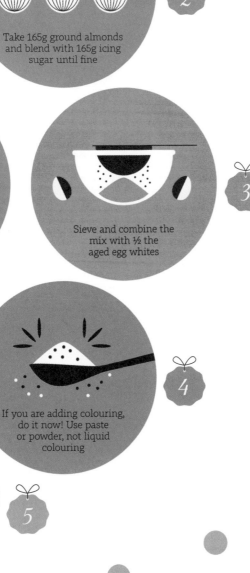

4

If you are adding colouring,
do it now! Use paste
or powder, not liquid
colouring

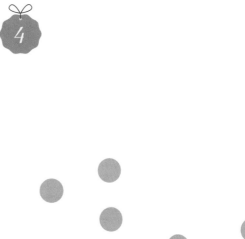

120°C

5

Bring 150g sugar and
50ml water to 120°C

—

PAVLOVA: AUSTRALIA'S PRIDE AND JOY (OR IS IT?)

I doubt Russian ballerina Anna Pavlova dreamed that her legacy would be a dessert fought over by the Antipodeans. But then again, pavlova is a really, really really good pudding.

Since her dancing heyday at the end of the 19th century, and early 20th century, Australia and New Zealand have battled over where the original pavlova was created. The former claim it was invented in the 1930s by Australian hotel chef Herbert Sachse in Perth, while New Zealand scholar Helen Leach believes, with some conviction, that the Kiwis had it first (name and invention). What is certain is that Anna visited both countries in the 1920s and that by the 1940s both were whipping up pavlova in her honour. Chicken or egg, either way, it's delicious and we should be thankful to that *en pointe* princess.

Too dry?
Crumble the meringue into chunks, combine with whipped cream and soft or stewed fruits into an English-style Eton Mess

MERINGUE MANTRA

1. Start with a squeaky clean bowl
2. Aged eggs are best (separated whites keep well in the fridge and freezer)
3. Add sugar after you've whisked the whites to a stiff peak
4. Store meringues in airtight containers at room temperature – the fridge will make them 'weep'

Too flat?
Stack your flat meringues into a tiered Pavlova with more cream, ice cream or Chantilly cream and fruits, in a French-style Vacherin dessert

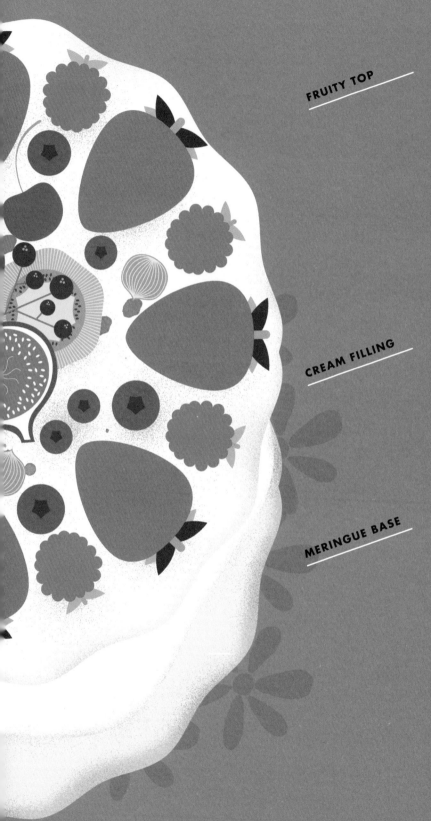

FRUITY TOP

Get creative with the toppings. Keep it traditional with tropical fruits such as passion fruit and mango or kiwi, or crown the cream with soft berries like strawberries, raspberries and blueberries. Sour fruits work really well against the sweet meringue, too – try stewed rhubarb and ginger or gooseberries and elderflower. Or mix it up completely with a salted caramel sauce and slices of banana, or shards of praline with grated dark chocolate

CREAM FILLING

Whip cream until dreamily 'just right', fluffy and cloud-like: too thin and it will run down the sides of your crisp meringue, too thick and it will start to resemble butter. The cream can be sweetened with icing sugar or flavoured with liqueurs, rose water or orange blossom water, hazelnut/chocolate spread, or citrus curds – just keep it light

MERINGUE BASE

The meringue should be a basic French meringue (i.e. whipped egg whites and sugar) but with the addition of a clear vinegar or lemon juice and cornflour to help produce a crispy outside shell and chewy, marshmallow-like centre when baked low and slow. You can also add vanilla essence, cocoa powder, ground nuts or coffee essence for a flavoured base, or make a brown sugar meringue instead. Either way, once the meringue has finished baking, leave it in the oven, with the door slightly ajar until it is completely cool and dry

TIRAMISU: LAYER CAKE

What dessert better promises a good time than the Venetian tiramisu, whose name literally means 'pick me up'. Incredibly though, despite its popularity at home and abroad, it was only created less than 50 years ago.

As ever, there is debate over who exactly invented this modern classic. Italian cookbooks, first publishing the recipe in the early 1980s, attribute it to pastry chef Loly Linguanotto of the Treviso restaurant Alle Beccherie but this family friendly recipe included no Marsala wine (which is now an essential component). Subsequently another pastry chef, Carminantonio Iannaccone, also from Treviso, claimed it was he who created the iconic dessert in 1969 from a collection of local, everyday ingredients: espresso, mascarpone, eggs, Marsala and sponge biscuits. And it is his alcoholic version that has become so popular around the world. Regardless it's a winner and easily replicated at home. It's all in the layers...

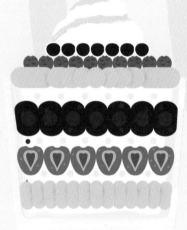

NO TRIFLING MATTER!

Across the Channel, Blighty has its own layered pudding, trifle, but with a far more longstanding history. The English created an early version of the traditional pudding with custard poured over alcohol-soaked bread, almost 400 years ago. The difference between tiramisu and trifle of course, is the inclusion of fruit and there are modern variations on the trifle theme that include everything from summer berries to mango, pineapple and spiced dried fruits

COCOA POWDER

Finish with a dusting of the dark stuff, although you can also experiment with milk, dark and white chocolate curls and shavings

MASCARPONE CREAM

This fresh Italian cream cheese is the key ingredient to a tiramisu and should authentically be enriched into a sweet mascarpone custard cream, similar to a zabaglione, with egg yolks, sugar, (sometimes) Marsala and beaten egg whites. Cheaters might ditch the eggs and lighten the mascarpone with double cream and Marsala

SOAKED SPONGE BISCUITS

The original recipe calls for ladyfinger or boudoir biscuits but as long as they are sweet, airy and crumbly with good potential for soaking up the coffee and alcohol mix, you're OK

MASCARPONE CREAM

Divide your cream into three even layers – or better yet, two fat ones

SOAKED SPONGE BISCUITS

A trial as old as time – how do you achieved soaked not soggy? An assertive plunge rather than a tentative dip in the liquid works best

CHOCOLATE

Cocoa powder or smattering of chocolate shavings between the layers if you please

MASCARPONE CREAM

You could leave out the Marsala in the cream, what with the booze in the soaked biscuits but... why would you?

SOAKED SPONGE BISCUITS

The bottom layer of biscuits is the foundation of a good tiramisu, so be sure to pack in plenty for a satisfying and supportive base. Each finger should be dipped in a mix of cold espresso (don't cut corners with instant coffee) and, if you're being classic, brandy or Marsala. You can go crazy though with orange-scented Grand Mariner, perhaps rum, or Tia Maria. Be careful with the liqueurs though – it should enhance not dominate

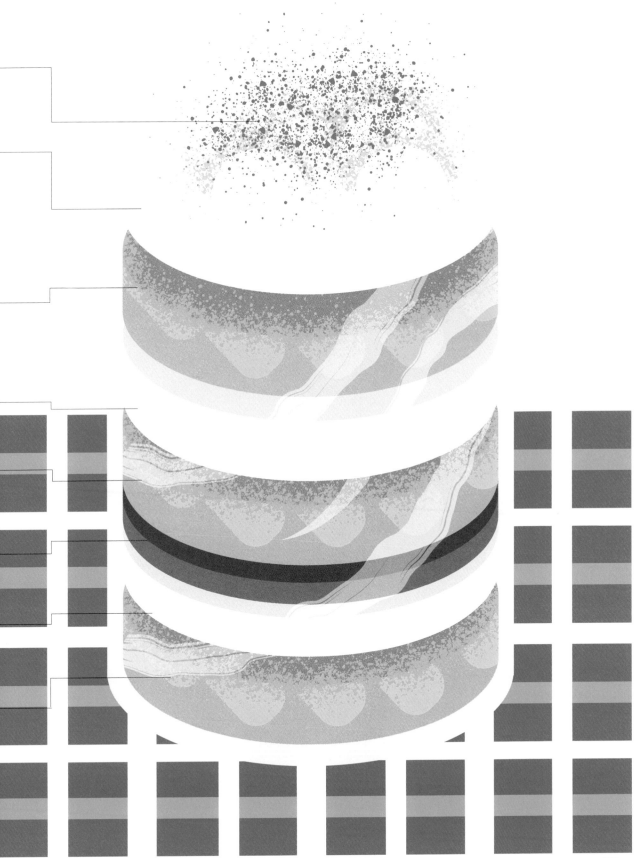

1. Add 9g instant yeast to 60ml warm water, stir, allow to get frothy. Add 250ml warm milk.

2. Place 650g plain flour, 1 tsp fine salt, 65g caster sugar in a separate bowl and rub together with 60g cold cubed unsalted butter until the mix resembles breadcrumbs. Stir in 1 beaten egg with a knife. Make a well in the mix.

3. Pour the liquid into the well, gently incorporate the dry ingredients until a ball of dough is formed.

4. Knead until smooth. Place in an oiled bowl, cover with a shower cap, and leave to prove in a warm place for 1 hour or until doubled in size.

5. Knock back the dough and roll out a rectangle to a thickness of 1cm between two sheets of baking parchment. Chill for 45 minutes.

6. Using a rolling pin, beat 250g cold unsalted butter in a rectangle, around 2/3 smaller than the dough rectangle. Fold the bottom third of the dough up, and the top third down, like a parcel. Tuck in the edges to seal, turn the dough by 90°.

7. Add sheet of parchment on top and gently roll the dough away from you to form another neat rectangle. Repeat the fold to make another parcel and chill for 20 minutes.

8. Repeat the fold and roll, twice, then take two cutters to create the ring shapes. Press the cutter down in one sharp movement, don't twist.

9. Place the doughnut rings on an oiled tray, cover, and leave to prove in a warm place overnight.

10. Bring a large pan of vegetable oil to 175°C and fry the doughnuts in batches until golden on all sides. Drain on kitchen paper and while still warm dunk in flavoured sugars.

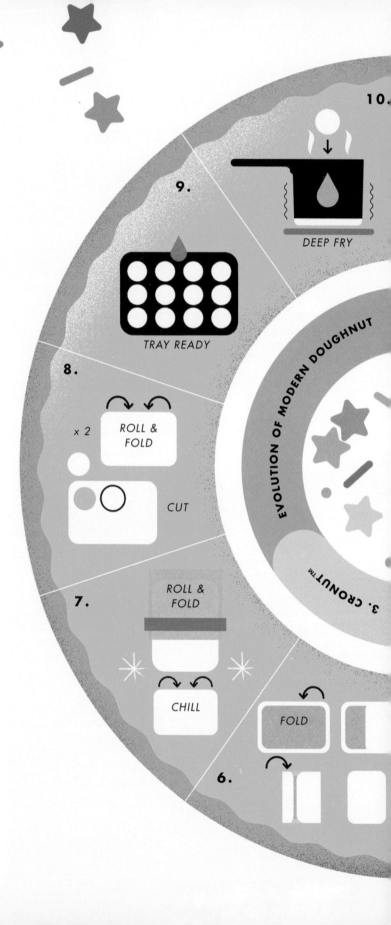

EVOLUTION OF MODERN DOUGHNUT

10.

9.

DEEP FRY

TRAY READY

8.

x 2   ROLL & FOLD

CUT

7.

ROLL & FOLD

CHILL

6.

FOLD

3. CRONUT™

DOUGHNUTS: WHOLE LOT OF FUN

Some foods are championed as 'super' because of their powers of good (packed full of vitamin this and that), but the doughnut is the ultimate foodie villain. The Darth Vader of the food world, naughty as they come, but universally loved. It helps that they're buttery, sweet, deep-fried, and dipped in sugar and stuffed with jam.

Although there are various types around the world – from tiny round Italian zeppole to the long and thin Spanish churro – the most famed and well loved are the American-style round and ring doughnuts.

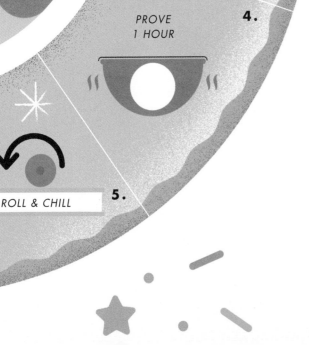

1.

WET MIX

2.

DRY MIX

3.

COMBINE WET AND DRY MIX

4.

PROVE 1 HOUR

5.

ROLL & CHILL

1. ROUND

2. RING

DECORATE

FILL
Pierce and fill round doughnuts with fruit jams and compotes, custard, chocolate ganache, or flavoured creams

DUST
While still warm, dip the doughnuts in caster sugar (plain or flavoured – cardamom, cinnamon, lavender, vanilla, etc) or dust in icing sugar

GLAZE
Mix icing sugar with milk or water until a thick liquid and pour over round or ring doughnuts. Leave to set

COOKIE: MONSTER

While you might imagine cookies – those sweetest of snacks that leave a trail of telltale crumbs in their wake – to be a recent addition to our culinary stable, they've actually been eaten for the past 300-odd years. It was in 1930, though, that the most iconic cookie of them all was invented.

There are different versions of the story that led to Ruth Wakefield, owner of the Toll House Inn in Whitman, Massachusetts, to create the holy grail of confectionery, the chocolate chip cookie. Some claim that when Wakefield found she was out of ordinary baking chocolate while preparing a batch of cookies she took a bar of Nestlé's semisweet chocolate and chopped it up finely expecting it to melt completely and flavour the whole cookie. Instead the chips remained whole, peppering the plain biscuit with delicious chunks. Wakefield herself claims it was a deliberate choice to introduce chips into a plain butterscotch nut cookie thus creating her now famous Toll House cookies. Either way, chocolate giant Nestlé bought the rights to the cookies and gave Ruth a lifetime's supply of Nestlé chocolate.

1. Cream together 100g caster sugar, 100g light Muscovado sugar and 125g unsalted butter (room temperature)

2. Beat in 1 medium egg and 1 egg yolk

3. Sieve 175g plain flour, ½ tsp bicarbonate of soda, ¼ tsp salt in a separate bowl

4. Mix the dry ingredients into the wet until a dough is formed

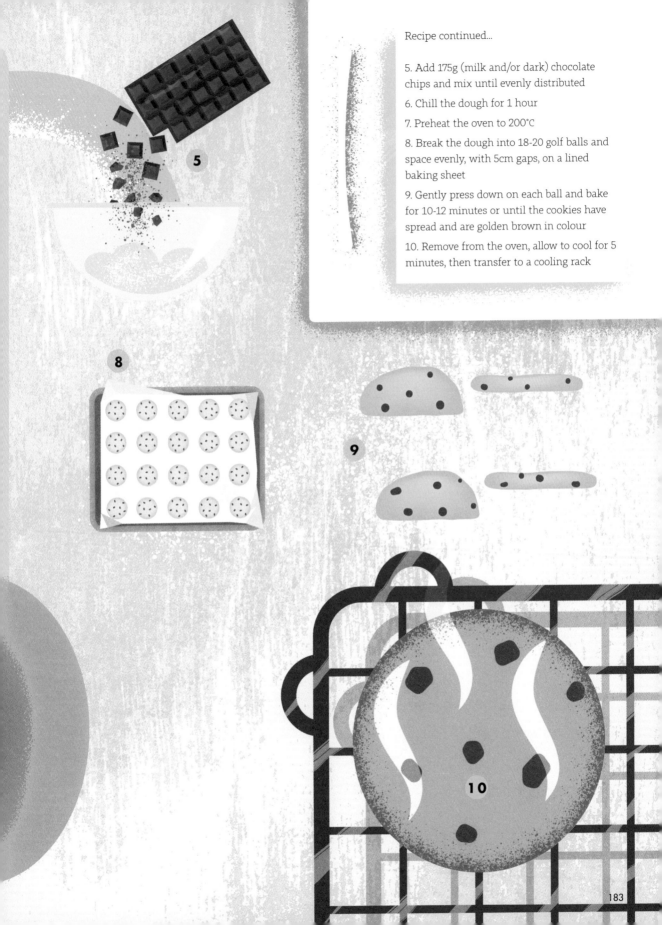

Recipe continued...

5. Add 175g (milk and/or dark) chocolate chips and mix until evenly distributed

6. Chill the dough for 1 hour

7. Preheat the oven to 200°C

8. Break the dough into 18-20 golf balls and space evenly, with 5cm gaps, on a lined baking sheet

9. Gently press down on each ball and bake for 10-12 minutes or until the cookies have spread and are golden brown in colour

10. Remove from the oven, allow to cool for 5 minutes, then transfer to a cooling rack

—

VICTORIA SPONGE: LET THEM EAT IT

If you are to learn the principles of one cake in your lifetime, Britain's classic teatime treat, the Victoria sponge, is the one. So simple and easily adapted, it is a must in any keen cook's culinary arsenal. Created in the mid-19th century, thanks to the invention of baking powder, and favoured by Queen Victoria, it is a creamed sponge sandwich cake and can be mastered by following a few simple tricks.

Start by preheating the oven to 180°C – this cake is quick, so you'll need it ready! Next, weigh out the ingredients. For two 20cm round tins, you need four eggs and the same weight (roughly 220g) of caster sugar, soft unsalted butter and self-raising flour. Melt a knob of butter leftover from the pack and, using kitchen paper, lightly grease the tins and line the bases with baking parchment. Make sure everything is at room temperature – any colder and you risk the mix curdling.

CHANGE IT UP:

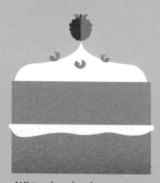

White chocolate buttercream and fresh blackberries, topped with white chocolate swirls

Elderberry jam filling, topped with vanilla sugar

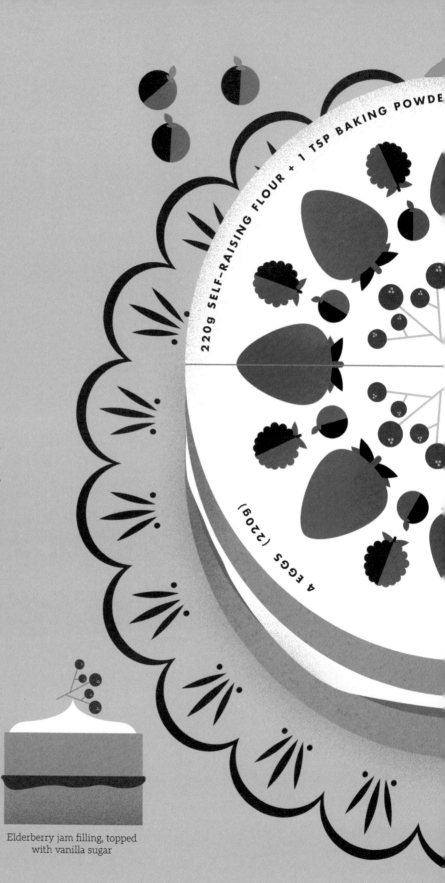

220g SELF-RAISING FLOUR + 1 TSP BAKING POWDER

4 EGGS (220g)

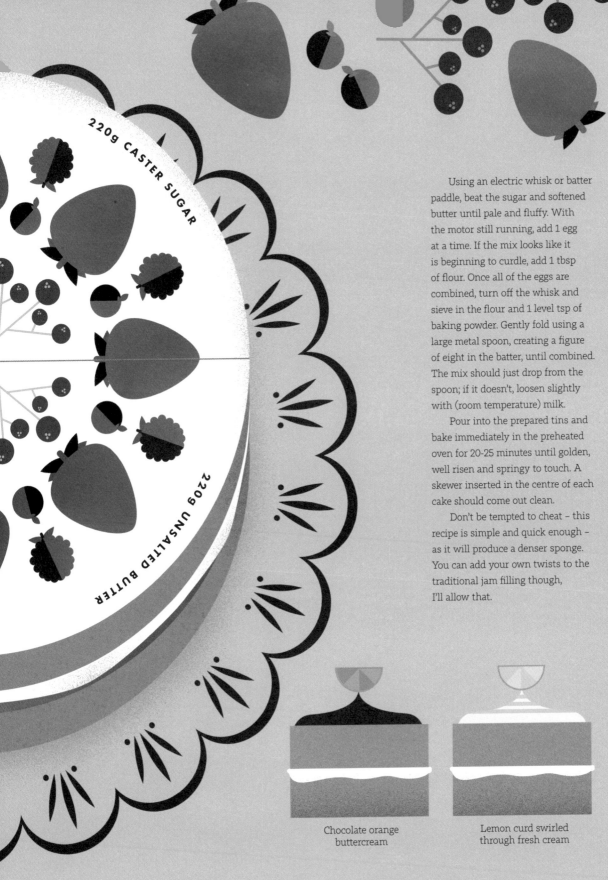

220g CASTER SUGAR

220g UNSALTED BUTTER

Using an electric whisk or batter paddle, beat the sugar and softened butter until pale and fluffy. With the motor still running, add 1 egg at a time. If the mix looks like it is beginning to curdle, add 1 tbsp of flour. Once all of the eggs are combined, turn off the whisk and sieve in the flour and 1 level tsp of baking powder. Gently fold using a large metal spoon, creating a figure of eight in the batter, until combined. The mix should just drop from the spoon; if it doesn't, loosen slightly with (room temperature) milk.

Pour into the prepared tins and bake immediately in the preheated oven for 20-25 minutes until golden, well risen and springy to touch. A skewer inserted in the centre of each cake should come out clean.

Don't be tempted to cheat – this recipe is simple and quick enough – as it will produce a denser sponge. You can add your own twists to the traditional jam filling though, I'll allow that.

Chocolate orange
buttercream

Lemon curd swirled
through fresh cream

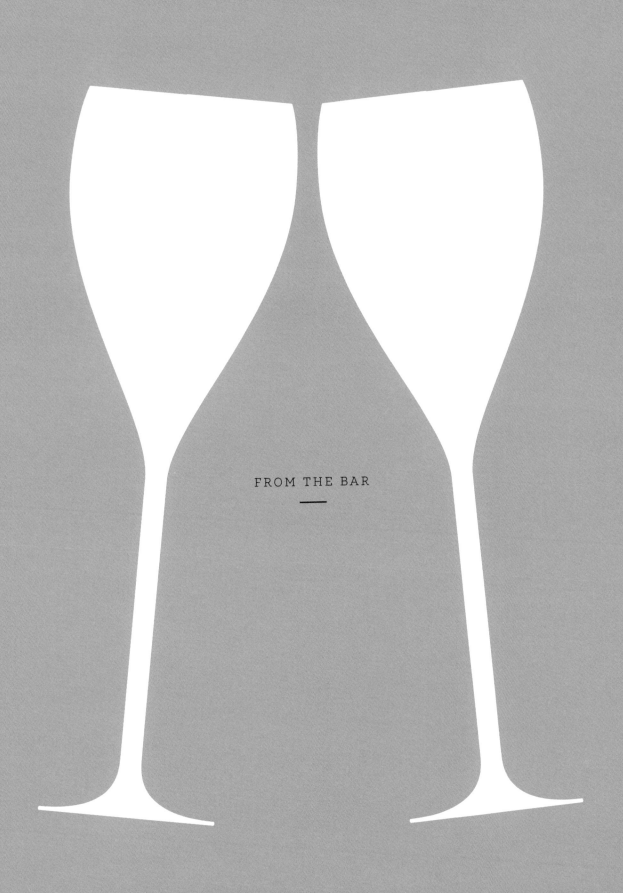

FROM THE BAR

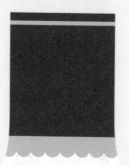

Cucumber
Elderflower
Lemongrass
Dandelion
Lemon
Gorse flower
Pineapple
Apple
Pear
Lime
Rosemary
Pine needle
Wild flower
Passion fruit
Orange
Mango
Ginger
Gooseberry
Rhubarb
Rose
Strawberry
Rosehip
Cranberry
Blood orange
Redcurrant
Pomegranate
Summer fruits
Raspberry
Plum
Blueberry
Blackcurrant
Blackberry
Fruits of the forest
Winter fruits

WHAT'S YOUR SQUEEZE?

Choose a blend of fruits, herbs and flower cordials for a delicious drink

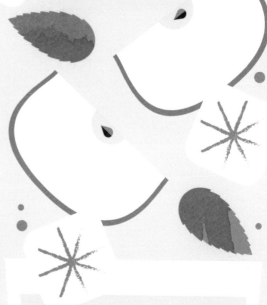

1/4

For the perfect mix, use one part cordial to four parts water

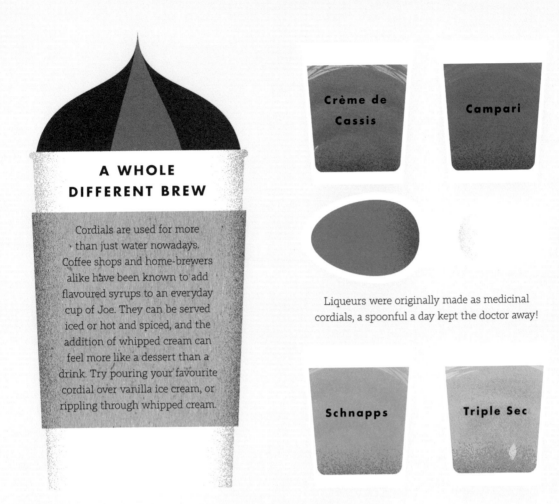

A WHOLE DIFFERENT BREW

Cordials are used for more than just water nowadays. Coffee shops and home-brewers alike have been known to add flavoured syrups to an everyday cup of Joe. They can be served iced or hot and spiced, and the addition of whipped cream can feel more like a dessert than a drink. Try pouring your favourite cordial over vanilla ice cream, or rippling through whipped cream.

Crème de Cassis

Campari

Liqueurs were originally made as medicinal cordials, a spoonful a day kept the doctor away!

Schnapps

Triple Sec

FROM THE BAR

—

CORDIAL: MAKING H$_2$0 HAPPY

While the term cordial nowadays might conjure up images of quintessential summer refreshment, the word can describe everything from a fruit concentrate to an alcoholic syrup. Early medieval cordials were in fact what we would call a liqueur today.

With a heavy dose of alcohol, one of the most popular medicines of the time, cordials were used to treat all kinds of ailments, especially those of the heart, nodding to the word's Latin origins ('cor' means heart in the classical language). Later, the Victorians created cordials from substances as strange as snake oil and as dangerous as opium, again with promises of health, rejuvenation and longevity.

The modern soft cordial is attributed to Lauchlin Rose who towards the end of the 19th century created lime cordial. Once again this was promoted on the grounds of health, probably due to the vitamin C content of the fruit that scurvy-avoiding sailors so famously took to sea. This was the first of many fruit-based concentrates such as lemon, orange, blackcurrant, cranberry or the more exotic pineapple and mango.

Recently there has been a boom in artisanal cordials, with more unusual flavours focusing on herbs, spices and floral notes – going back to the roots of cordial making which saw the whole garden explored for its infusion potential. Marketed as much to adults as water-loathing children, these have become a popular alternative for the designated driver with varieties such as elderflower becoming instant classics.

KNOW YOUR TEA LEAVES

WHITE
Try: Silver Needle Tea
Unfermented (often young) tea leaves and buds, which are left to wither and dry in the sun. Packed with antioxidants, low in caffeine, subtle and elegant in flavour, and best brewed in hot, not boiling water

OOLONG
Try: Wuyi Oolong
The next stage of processing, between green and black tea, oolong's large leaves are bruised once picked and allowed to dry and semi-ferment (different tea makers and countries will have different times for this), and then pan-fired. The flavour will vary depending on the level of oxidation and roasting but can range from fruity and floral, to spicy and toasted

HERBAL
Try: Fresh Mint
For those looking for caffeine-free teas there are thousands of alternatives – where herbs, fruits and spices are infused in boiling water. From simple fresh mint tea, as favoured by the Moroccans, to soothing chamomile or healing lemon peel and root ginger

GREEN
Try: Dragon Well
Unoxidised leaves that are heated once picked (either in a wok, or by steaming) to kill the enzymes that cause the oxidation process, then rolled. Around 80% is produced in China and it is the go-to drink for the health conscious. Less is more when it comes to brewing if you want to avoid a bitter flavour, go for 1-2 minutes in hot, not boiling water

BLACK
Try: English Breakfast
The most processed of all teas, black tea is fully fermented, then fired, to get its distinctively strong colour, aroma and taste. Best brewed in boiling water and essential to a classic English afternoon tea

PU-ERH
Aged black tea from the Chinese province, Yunnan with a complex, rich flavour. Can be raw (green) or cooked (black) and left loose or compressed

MATCHA
Shade-grown tea that is ground into a powder and used in ritualistic Japanese tea ceremonies and increasingly as a flavouring for foods. Favoured for its health properties (1 cup of matcha is said to have as many antioxidants as 10 cups of green tea), as you are consuming the whole leaf, rather than just the brewed water

ROOIBOS
Not strictly a tea at all, as not from the Camellia Sinensis plant – this red tea is from the South African bush of the same name. The leaves are harvested and bruised, sprayed with water, allowed to ferment, and then dried in the sun

FLAVOURED
Try: Chai tea
Green and black teas are often flavoured or infused with other ingredients, from citrus fruit (Earl Grey is black tea flavoured with bergamot) and flowers (green tea is often paired with aromatic jasmine petals) to spice (chai black tea can include everything from cinnamon and cardamom to peppercorns). Tea can also be smoked, as in lapsang souchong

TEA: TOTAL

Can't sleep? Make a cup of tea. Upset? Put the kettle on. Want to procrastinate from your work? Have a tea break. If you pick green, it's even said to help with weight loss. So, what is this magical 'tea'?

Real tea, whether white, green or black, from China, Japan or India, is made from the leaves of the evergreen shrub, Camellia Sinensis. It was first discovered some 5,000 years ago in China and is now essential to the economies of numerous countries around the world. Like wine, the terrior where it's grown influences its final flavour, along with the way it is processed.

Bearing this in mind, the best teas are loose leaf

(cheap teabags can literally just be the tea 'dust') and look out for single estate teas, made from one maker's 'garden' rather than a blend from various estates. The temperature and quality of water will also make a difference to the final brew (contrary to habit, boiling water isn't always best), along with the amount of time you leave it to steep. If you're buying from a good tea merchant they'll be able to advise how best to make each individual tea. From here, you can take it black, or with milk (or even butter as in Tibet), add sugar or another form of sweetener, and serve it hot or cold. Better yet, serve it with a slice of cake.

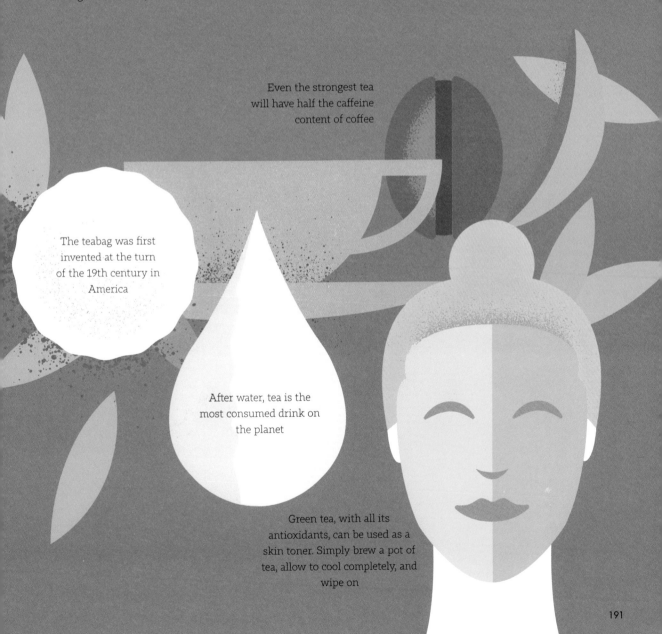

Even the strongest tea will have half the caffeine content of coffee

The teabag was first invented at the turn of the 19th century in America

After water, tea is the most consumed drink on the planet

Green tea, with all its antioxidants, can be used as a skin toner. Simply brew a pot of tea, allow to cool completely, and wipe on

COFFEE: A DAILY GRIND

As one of the most traded commodities, second only to oil, and one of the most consumed beverages in the entire world, coffee is kind of a big deal. It's the backbone of American sitcoms, the fuel of commuters and the promising end to a date. The good ol' cup of Joe could be the subject for a book in itself.

It's grown in more than 60 countries, the majority of which are within 1,000 miles of the equator in the 'bean belt'. The coffee tree bears deep red fruits, cherries, which are just over 1cm long and each contain two green beans. It takes 42 precious beans to make one espresso, which means a hell of a lot of beans need to be harvested for the two billion or so cups of coffee that are drunk around the world every single day.

Once the two main types of beans are harvested – Arabica, which accounts for 60% of world production, and Robusta – they then need to be roasted. It's this process that brings out the deep flavours and aromas that we've all become so addicted to. The beans stale from the minute they are picked but even more so after roasting and so, after a brief maturation period (around a week is ideal), should be ground in small batches.

Then all manner of magic can happen. Drip brew, cold press, percolate or steep; add water (filtered, around 91-96°C preferably), milk or sugar (although, most baristas worth their Arabica will say to skip both), butter (the latest craze in the US), eggs (really), syrups, spice, and more, and the world is your Java.

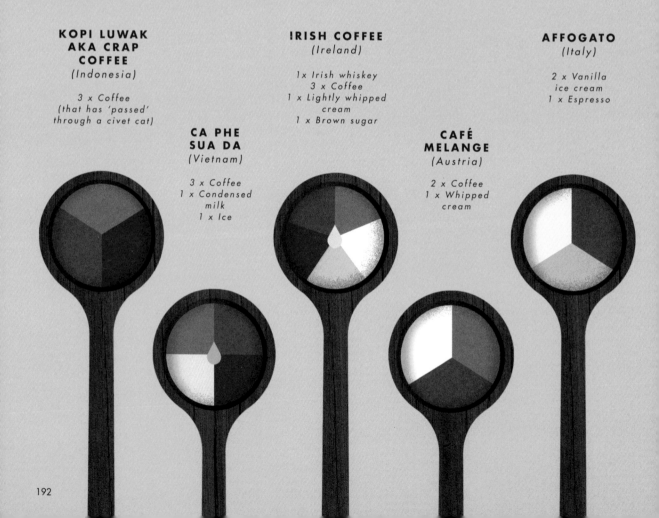

KOPI LUWAK AKA CRAP COFFEE
(Indonesia)

3 x Coffee
(that has 'passed' through a civet cat)

IRISH COFFEE
(Ireland)

1x Irish whiskey
3 x Coffee
1 x Lightly whipped cream
1 x Brown sugar

AFFOGATO
(Italy)

2 x Vanilla ice cream
1 x Espresso

CA PHE SUA DA
(Vietnam)

3 x Coffee
1 x Condensed milk
1 x Ice

CAFÉ MELANGE
(Austria)

2 x Coffee
1 x Whipped cream

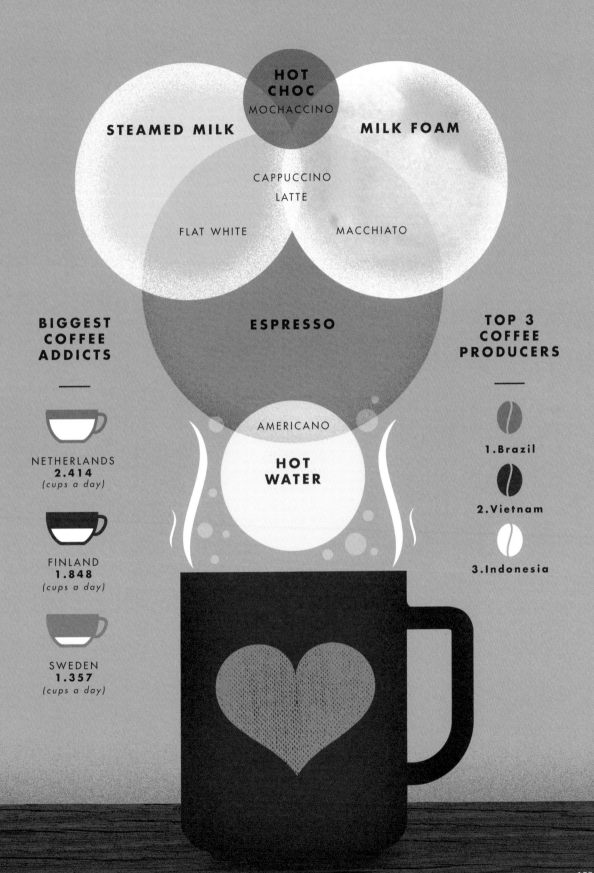

HOT
CHOC
MOCHACCINO

STEAMED MILK

MILK FOAM

CAPPUCCINO
LATTE

FLAT WHITE

MACCHIATO

ESPRESSO

BIGGEST
COFFEE
ADDICTS

NETHERLANDS
2.414
(cups a day)

FINLAND
1.848
(cups a day)

SWEDEN
1.357
(cups a day)

AMERICANO

HOT
WATER

TOP 3
COFFEE
PRODUCERS

1.Brazil

2.Vietnam

3.Indonesia

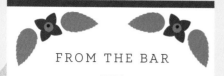

FROM THE BAR

—

BITTERS: THE TRUTH

Just as a pinch of salt or a spoonful of sugar can help enliven a meal, the tiniest drop of bitters can seriously shift gears in a cocktail, cranking it from 'nice' to a serious taste experience. So what is this little magic potion?

Made from a strong, alcoholic base, and infused with herbs and spices, they were originally used for medicinal purposes or as a digestive aid. The alcohol, a common treatment for various ailments, released the herbs' aromas, flavours and essential oils, acted as a preservative and helped take the edge off some of the extreme bitterness.

The most famous survivor, and a regular feature in cocktail bars across the world, is Angostura Bitters. Named after its Venezuelan town of origin, it was invented by German doctor Johann Gottlieb Benjamin Siegert as a medicinal tonic for seasickness and stomach complaints. The tonic made its way over to European shores via sailors and their ships and by 1850 it was being distributed the world over. It is now used to flavour food and drink, and even as a mosquito repellent by some, and is famed for its oversized label (the result of laidback Caribbean attitudes – and it stuck). It is also, perhaps surprisingly, not bitter – it is merely used as an aromatic, to temper, marry and enhance the ingredients it shares glass space with.

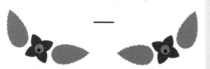

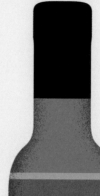

ANGOSTURA

Distilled in Trinidad and still made to the original secret recipe from 1824. A classic cocktail ingredient, particularly in a Manhattan and Old Fashioned and is said to include over 40 flavours including clove, anise, gentian, cardamom, nutmeg and cinnamon

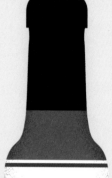

REGAN'S

Makers of Orange Bitters No.6, a less sweet but spicier citrus bitter excellent in cocktails like the Martinez, or any rum- or Scotch-based cocktails

PEYCHAUD'S

Dating back to New Orleans in 1838 this floral, lighter bitters includes gentian and anise. Famously good in a Sazerac

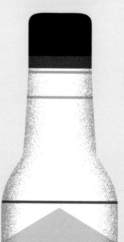

FEE BROTHERS

American company with everything from Aztec Chocolate and Black Walnut to Gin Barrel-Aged Orange, Grapefruit and Rhubarb on its books

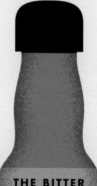

THE BITTER TRUTH

Created by German bartenders Stephan Berg and Alexander Hauck. The most respected is the Bitterman's range with highlights including orange, celery, or the spicy Mexican-inspired Xocolatl Mole bitters

MAKE YOUR OWN

Experiment with infusing high-proof, neutral alcohol (like vodka) with a 'bittering agent' – that could be anything from chillies to coffee, to more unusual ingredients like wormword. Allow to infuse for several weeks, then strain

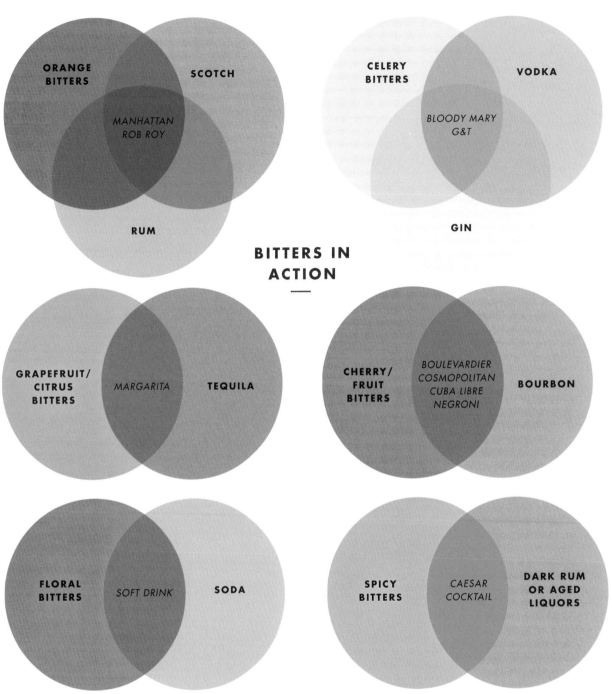

BITTERS IN ACTION

ORANGE BITTERS · **SCOTCH** · **RUM**
MANHATTAN / ROB ROY

CELERY BITTERS · **VODKA** · **GIN**
BLOODY MARY / G&T

GRAPEFRUIT/ CITRUS BITTERS · **TEQUILA**
MARGARITA

CHERRY/ FRUIT BITTERS · **BOURBON**
BOULEVARDIER / COSMOPOLITAN / CUBA LIBRE / NEGRONI

FLORAL BITTERS · **SODA**
SOFT DRINK

SPICY BITTERS · **DARK RUM OR AGED LIQUORS**
CAESAR COCKTAIL

SWEDISH BITTERS

The most famous of the digestive bitters, Swedish Bitters reputedly date back to the time of the Renaissance physician and occultist Paracelsus, and were rediscovered by Swedish medics in the 18th century. In the 20th century they were popularised by the books of Austrian herbalist, Maria Treben and were said to help digestion by stimulating stomach acid, alongside loftier claims to cure more serious illnesses. Main ingredients include: Angelica root, carline thistle root, camphor, manna, myrrh, saffron, rhubarb root, senna, theriac Venetian and zedoary root.

BEER: PINT OF

Beer is bitter and comes in a pint glass, right? Well, yes, but there are two main types of beer – ale and lager – and numerous different styles that are produced around the world that are ready and waiting to be enjoyed.

The main differences between the two are the yeast and temperature that are used in the brewing process. Ale, which is thought to be the oldest beer, uses top-fermenting yeast, which rises to the top and eventually sinks, and is capable of producing stronger, more complex beers. It is also generally brewed at warmer temperatures (between 18–24°C). Lager, meanwhile, likes it cool at around 8–12°C, and uses bottom-fermenting yeast for longer, producing a crisp, clear beer. Both are made from the same basic ingredients: water, grain (usually barley), yeast and hops but brewers can add any ingredients they like, from sugar or honey, to wheat and rye, fruit, herbs, spices and even oysters.

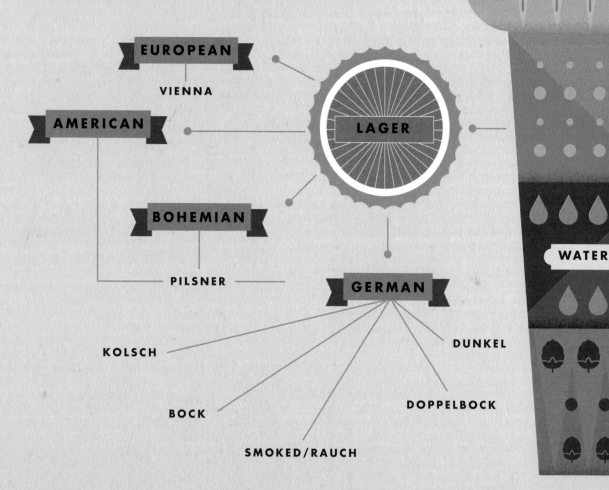

EUROPEAN

VIENNA

AMERICAN

LAGER

BOHEMIAN

PILSNER

GERMAN

KOLSCH

DUNKEL

BOCK

DOPPELBOCK

SMOKED/RAUCH

GRAIN

WATER

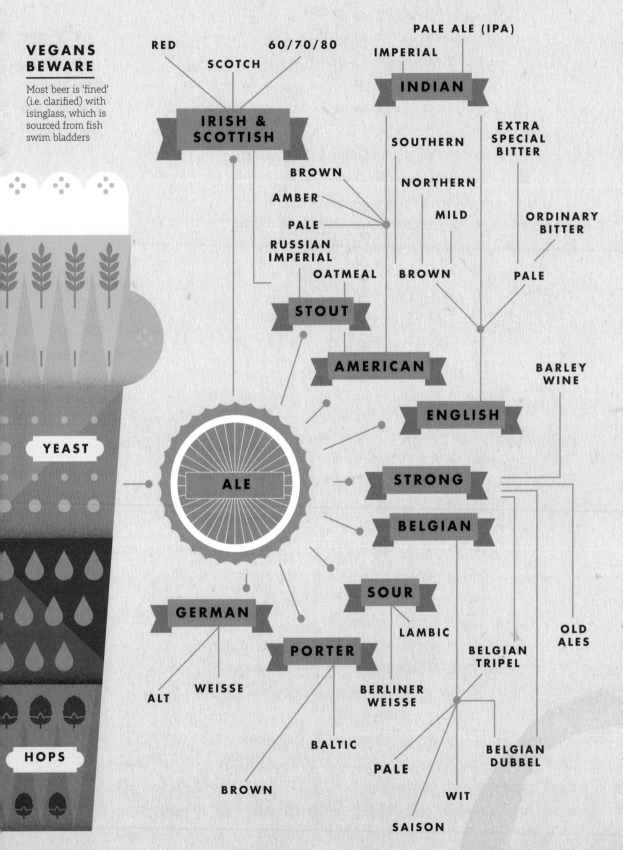

VEGANS BEWARE

Most beer is 'fined' (i.e. clarified) with isinglass, which is sourced from fish swim bladders

RED

SCOTCH

60/70/80

PALE ALE (IPA)

IMPERIAL

INDIAN

IRISH & SCOTTISH

EXTRA SPECIAL BITTER

SOUTHERN

BROWN

NORTHERN

ORDINARY BITTER

AMBER

MILD

PALE

RUSSIAN IMPERIAL

OATMEAL

BROWN

PALE

STOUT

AMERICAN

BARLEY WINE

ENGLISH

YEAST

ALE

STRONG

BELGIAN

OLD ALES

SOUR

GERMAN

LAMBIC

BELGIAN TRIPEL

PORTER

ALT

WEISSE

BERLINER WEISSE

BELGIAN DUBBEL

BALTIC

PALE

HOPS

BROWN

WIT

SAISON

197

CIDER: THE RISE AND RISE

The drink we know as cider starts with apples. In North America and much of Canada it refers to a sweet apple soft drink – unfermented and unfiltered – while in Europe it's an alcoholic beverage that can be sweet or dry, sparkling or still, clear or cloudy – but always with a distinctive flavour of the cider apples.

PERRY GOOD

Perry is a similar drink to cider but made with pears instead of cider apples. Different flavours and fruits can be added to cider but often these are inferior drinks made with concentrates

MORE THAN A DRINK

Cider might be a drink but it is great in cooking too. Pour into white meat – from chicken pieces or pork, to pheasant and bacon – and reduce down for sauces with mustard and cream. Add to steaming mussels, instead of wine, or swap sparkling water or beer in batters for deep-frying with a sparkling cider

PAY DAY

During the 18th century orchard owners in the UK, particularly the South West, which is famed for its cider-making heritage, used to pay part of its workers' wages with the hard stuff

ICE IS NICE

In the last decade cider drinking has changed. It's become an essential part of summer drinking and thanks to marketing campaigns by the big producers, there is a new trend to drink sparkling ciders over ice

SWEET   BITTERSWEET   BITTERSHARP   SHARP

APPLE WATCH

Most cider makers use a blend of cider apples to produce the perfect balance of sweetness, acidity, tannins (which affect the mouthfeel) and juice yield. There are thought to be hundreds of cider apple cultivars but in reality only around a dozen or so (such as Dabinett or Michelin) are used regularly by the commercial producers. Don't even think about eating these fruits though – they're tough and sour, and best kept for drinking only!

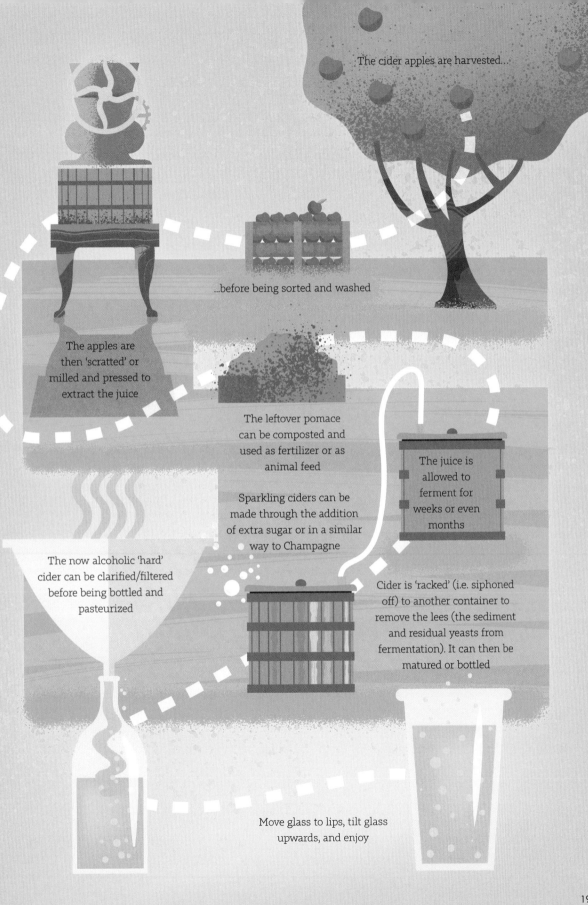

The cider apples are harvested...

...before being sorted and washed

The apples are then 'scratted' or milled and pressed to extract the juice

The leftover pomace can be composted and used as fertilizer or as animal feed

Sparkling ciders can be made through the addition of extra sugar or in a similar way to Champagne

The juice is allowed to ferment for weeks or even months

The now alcoholic 'hard' cider can be clarified/filtered before being bottled and pasteurized

Cider is 'racked' (i.e. siphoned off) to another container to remove the lees (the sediment and residual yeasts from fermentation). It can then be matured or bottled

Move glass to lips, tilt glass upwards, and enjoy

**1 GLASS =
1 MILLION BUBBLES**

*Champagne should be bright,
crystal clear and range in
colour according to its age*

*Should be poured
at an angle of
45° from the
bottle and
7-10°C
cold*

*Look out for
streams of
bubbles rising
up to the
'mousse'*

FROM THE BAR

—

CHAMPAGNE:
FINE FIZZ

No other drink in the world says
'celebration' quite like Champagne. Native to
Northern France, only 60 miles east of Paris,
Champagne is a sparkling wine from the region of
the same name and is home to 319 wine-making
villages and more than 15,000 wine growers.

Traditionally, Champagne is made of a blend of
white and red wine grapes – Pinot Noir, Pinot
Meunier and Chardonnay. While still wine is the
result of fermentation, Champagne's bubbles, like
most sparkling wines, are the product of a second
fermentation through the addition of yeast
and sugar. Since 1936 the famous fizz has been
awarded an AOC (Appellation d'Origine contrôlée)
thanks to its unique terroir, with its northerly
latitude, cool climate and chalky soils.

Other sparkling wines are available around the
world, from Spain's Cava and Italy's Prosecco
to Germany's Deutscher Sekt. And, you can
find increasingly good sparkling wines from
England, Brazil, Australasia and South Africa too.
It's thought that every two seconds a bottle of
Champagne is popped around the world.

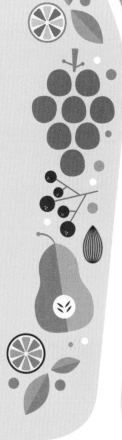

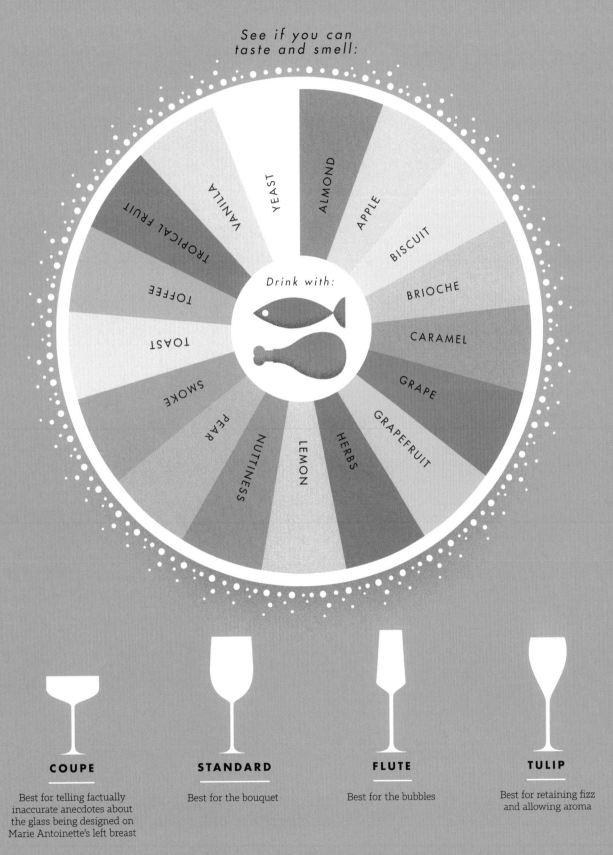

See if you can
taste and smell:

YEAST
ALMOND
APPLE
BISCUIT
BRIOCHE
CARAMEL
GRAPE
GRAPEFRUIT
HERBS
LEMON
NUTTINESS
PEAR
SMOKE
TOAST
TOFFEE
TROPICAL FRUIT
VANILLA

Drink with:

COUPE

Best for telling factually
inaccurate anecdotes about
the glass being designed on
Marie Antoinette's left breast

STANDARD

Best for the bouquet

FLUTE

Best for the bubbles

TULIP

Best for retaining fizz
and allowing aroma

WINE: GRAPE EXPECTATIONS

There is perhaps no other alcoholic drink so closely associated with the food we eat than wine. We've been drinking it for thousands of years and it has become more important than ever. Choosing the right wine with your meal will enhance the flavours of a dish.

However, the world of wine is a vast and seemingly complicated one. With so much terminology to master, an overwhelming selection to choose from and inherent snobbery of what's 'right or wrong' it can be hard to know where to start. So let's learn the basics and remember: there are always exceptions to the rules!

SERVE YOUR WINE

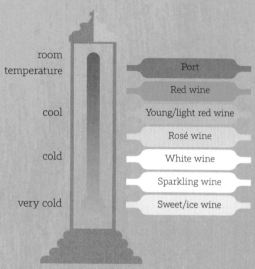

room temperature	Port
	Red wine
cool	Young/light red wine
	Rosé wine
cold	White wine
	Sparkling wine
very cold	Sweet/ice wine

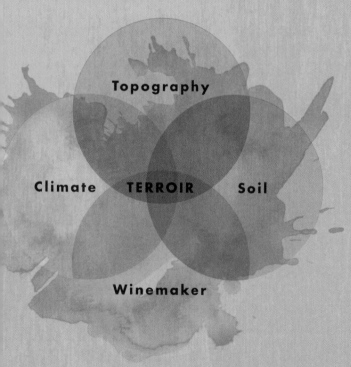

Topography

Climate **TERROIR** Soil

Winemaker

HOW TO TASTE (AND ENJOY) YOUR WINE AS A NON-PROFESSIONAL

1. Keeping the base of the glass flat on the table, swirl the wine in the glass and take a good sniff. There are thousands of aromas to detect but the common types of scents include floral, herbal, spicy and vegetal notes. Vanilla, chocolate and coffee smells are often imparted by the barrel the wine is aged in, while other varieties, such as the French sweet wine Sauternes, might smell of honey thanks to the noble rot on the vines before the grapes are pressed. Don't skip this stage – the smell is essential to the flavour of the wine

2. Professionals will sip, and suck the wine into the back of the mouth to fully aerate and spread the wine around the whole mouth but if you're just at home a simple mouthful will do. Appreciate the flavours (from the taste and smell) at the beginning, middle and end, and think about whether the wine is sweet, dry, acidic, astringent with tannins, intense, how alcoholic it is, and how long the taste lingers. A good wine will be balanced but complex. Being able to detect flavour notes will help if you are keen to complement your drink to your dinner i.e. acidic wines like fatty foods

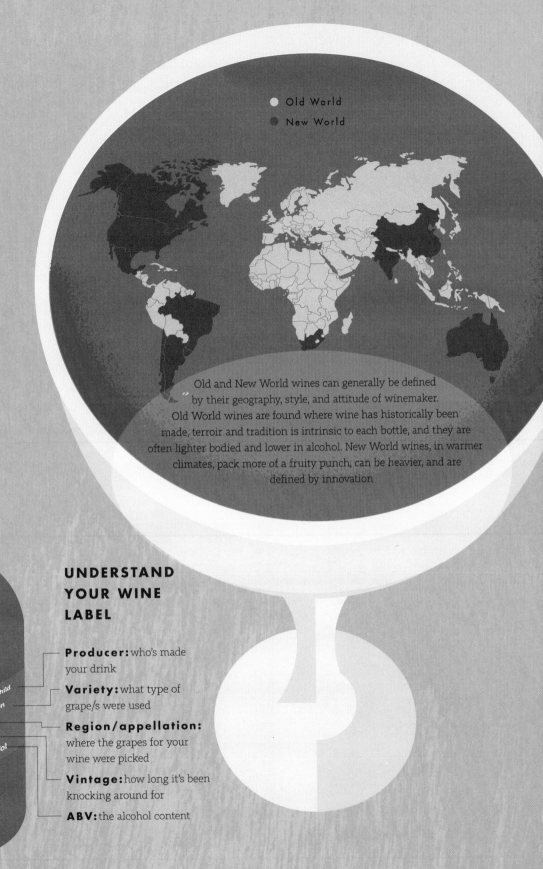

Old World

New World

Old and New World wines can generally be defined
by their geography, style, and attitude of winemaker.
Old World wines are found where wine has historically been
made, terroir and tradition is intrinsic to each bottle, and they are
often lighter bodied and lower in alcohol. New World wines, in warmer
climates, pack more of a fruity punch, can be heavier, and are
defined by innovation

UNDERSTAND YOUR WINE LABEL

Château Lafite Rothschild

Cabernet Sauvignon

Pauillac

2000

12.5% Vol

Producer: who's made your drink

Variety: what type of grape/s were used

Region/appellation: where the grapes for your wine were picked

Vintage: how long it's been knocking around for

ABV: the alcohol content

—

COCKTAILS: A DIRTY DOZEN

Just as any good meal is balanced – sweet and sour, salty and bitter – a cocktail requires considered measurement. At its most traditional, a mix of spirit, sugar, water (through ice) and bitters, the modern cocktail is constantly evolving. But always, the art of imbibing is about theatre and pleasure, whether made at home or consumed at the hands of others. These are the classic ingredients for some of the world's most celebrated cocktails but as with any recipe, there's always a little room for interpretation. Experiment with fruit purées in a Bellini (I actually prefer lychee or raspberry); or exchange the booze in a sour (amaretto is a winner), for example.

You will need:
Cocktail shaker (with strainer)
muddler, bar spoon & lots of ice

—

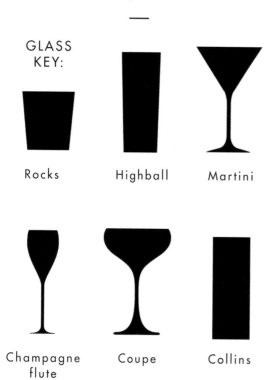

GLASS KEY:

Rocks

Highball

Martini

Champagne flute

Coupe

Collins

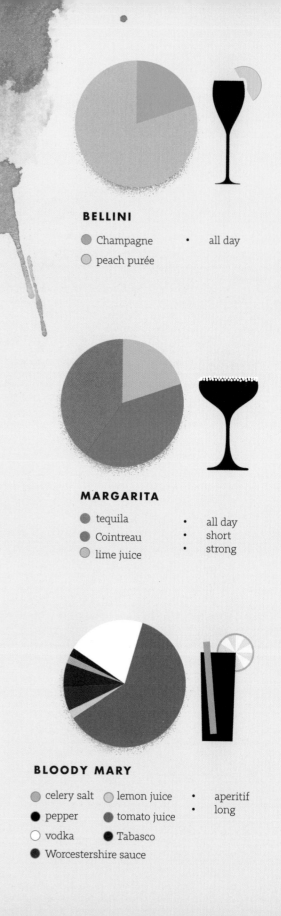

BELLINI
- Champagne
- peach purée
- all day

MARGARITA
- tequila
- Cointreau
- lime juice
- all day
- short
- strong

BLOODY MARY
- celery salt
- pepper
- vodka
- Worcestershire sauce
- lemon juice
- tomato juice
- Tabasco
- aperitif
- long

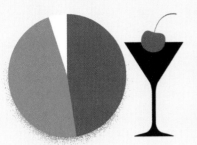 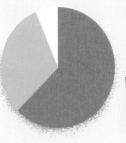 

MANHATTAN

- ● bourbon
- ○ bitters
- ● sweet vermouth

- · aperitif
- · short
- · strong

NEGRONI

- ● gin
- ● Campari
- ● sweet vermouth

- · aperitif
- · short
- · strong

CAIPIRINHA

- ● cachaça
- ○ sugar
- ● lime (cut into segments)

- · aperitif
- · short
- · strong

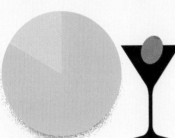 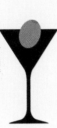 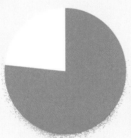 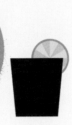 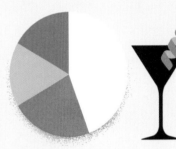

MARTINI

- ● gin
- ● dry vermouth

- · aperitif
- · strong

OLD FASHIONED

- ● bourbon
- ○ bitters
- ○ sugar cube

- · digestif
- · short
- · strong

COSMOPOLITAN

- ● lime juice
- ● Cointreau
- ○ citrus vodka
- ● cranberry juice

- · all day
- · long

 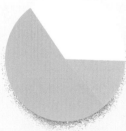 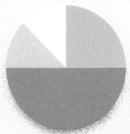 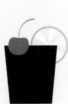 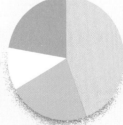 

TOM COLLINS

- ● gin
- ● lemon juice
- ○ bitters
- ○ sugar syrup

- · all day
- · long

WHISKY SOUR

- ● whisky
- ● egg white
- ○ sugar syrup
- ● lemon juice

- · all day
- · short

MOJITO

- ● lime juice
- ● white rum
- ○ sugar syrup
- ● mint leaves

- · all day
- · long

GIN: MOTHER'S RUIN

Passed aside as a cheap, easy to make spirit, it's only in the last five years that we've truly seen its renaissance.

Essentially a flavoured spirit, gin starts life as neutral, clear alcohol, made from grain (like vodka) which is then redistilled with natural botanicals, whose job is to impart unique flavours and aromas. As a drink, it's inspired by the sweeter, juniper-flavoured Dutch genever. It's thought that it came to British shores with soldiers around the 17th century, and accelerated in popularity thanks to the Dutch king at the time, William of Orange.

There are two main types of gin to look out for. Compound gin is made by adding natural extracts or botanicals to a neutral spirit (these tend to be cheaper to make and often inferior), while distilled gin is, as it sounds, made by redistilling with the botanicals. London Dry, is one such example of the latter (although interestingly can be made anywhere in the world). There is a new breed of gins now being made too, called New Western Dry, which sees juniper take a backseat to its fellow botanicals. And while the ingredients of many modern bottles might read like the shopping list for a witch's broth, the greater the number of botanicals doesn't necessarily mean the greater the gin. It's an art form; you just need to find the right style for you.

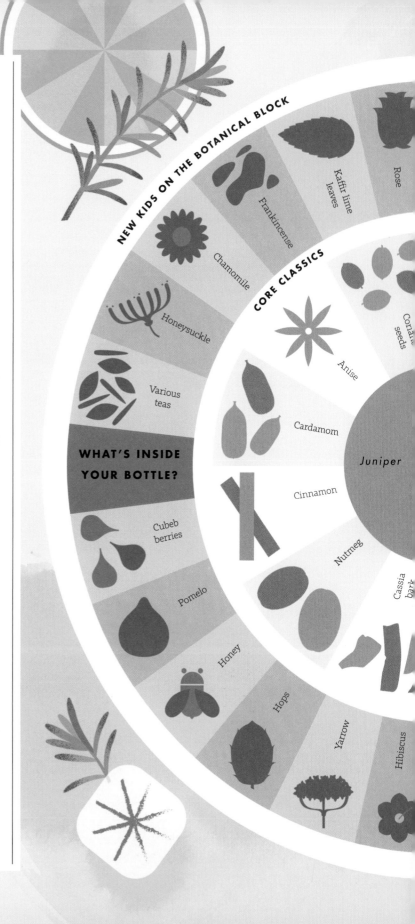

NEW KIDS ON THE BOTANICAL BLOCK

Frankincense

Kaffir lime leaves

Rose

Chamomile

CORE CLASSICS

Honeysuckle

Anise

Coriander seeds

Various teas

Cardamom

Juniper

WHAT'S INSIDE YOUR BOTTLE?

Cinnamon

Cubeb berries

Nutmeg

Cassia bark

Pomelo

Honey

Hops

Yarrow

Hibiscus

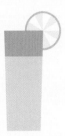

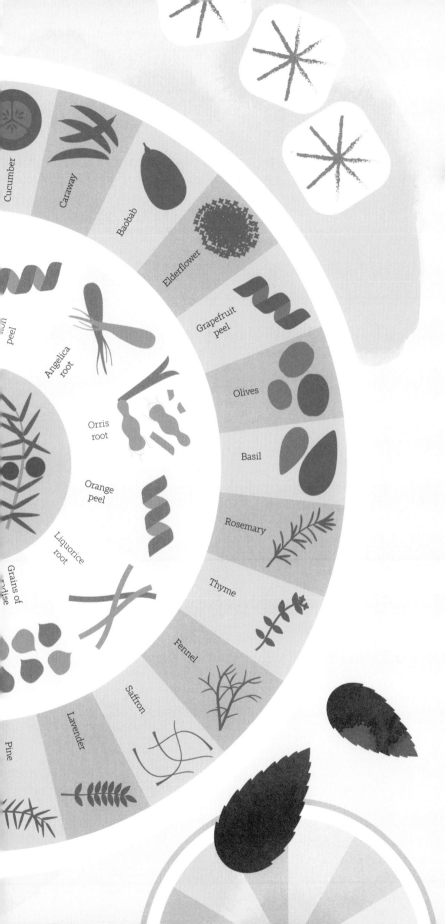

Cucumber

Caraway

Baobab

Elderflower

Grapefruit peel

...peel

Angelica root

Orris root

Orange peel

Olives

Basil

Rosemary

Liquorice root

Thyme

Grains of ...rise

Fennel

Saffron

Lavender

Pine

RAMOS GIN FIZZ

2 msr gin
1 msr lemon juice
½ msr lime juice
½ msr sugar syrup
⅛ msr orange flower water
1 msr egg white
1 msr double cream
Garnish: slice of lemon
Glass: highball

BRAMBLE

2 msr gin
½ msr blackberry liqueur
1 msr lemon juice
½ msr sugar syrup
Garnish: blackberries
Glass: rocks

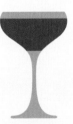

AVIATION

2 msr gin
½ msr crème de violette
⅛ msr cherry liqueur
1 msr lemon juice
Garnish: none
Glass: coupe

—

WHISKY: A WEE DRAM

Fine wine might steal all the limelight when it comes to intoxicating liquids but with quality and sophistication so dependent on the process, blend and bottling of the individual distilleries, whisky can be just as interesting and rewarding.

Those who enjoy the amber nectar often disagree over what makes the perfect sup. From the supply and taste of the water used, to the cask they are laid to rest in, each element in the whisky-making practice has a profound effect on the overall quality, design and taste.

What's not in contention, though, are the three necessary elements needed to craft a single malt whisky: water, malted barley and yeast. It's then the subtle use of peat and oak, which differs depending on where it's made.

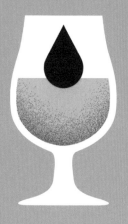

TIPS FOR YOUR TIPPLE

1. Although whisky is associated with the short tumbler some suggest this is not ideal for tasting – use a tulip-shaped glass with a reasonable sized bowl instead

2. Ice might be the natural go-to but it can inhibit the aroma

and flavour of the whisky, making it harder to pick up the finer notes

3. A small amount of water, instead, is recommended to help open up the flavours and aroma of your dram, but think drops not splashes

FROM GRAIN TO GLASS

1.MALTING

Barley grains are steeped in water and allowed to partially germinate in order to convert the barley starch to malt sugars that can be fermented into alcohol. Traditionally this was done by spreading the grain on a malting floor

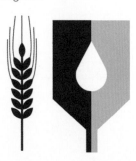

2.MASHING

The malt is milled into flour, which in turn is mixed with hot water into a mash. Water of varying temperatures is run through the mash three times to extract a sugar solution, known as a 'wort'

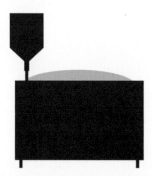

3.FERMENTATION

The wort is mixed with yeast and allowed to ferment into alcohol

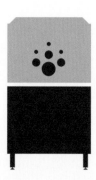

SCOTCH WHISKEY

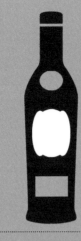

Historically, the Scots are considered the big boys in the single malt whisky world. They'll tell you this is due to the natural water springs in their mountains. The effects of mining have also fed into the earth, seeping into the natural bogs and wet marshlands that the distilleries use for peat, affecting the taste of the malt, and therefore the whisky. It's because of all this that it can only be labelled Scotch if it is 100% made in Scotland

BOURBON

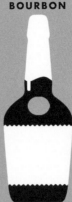

From the desperation of dirt-poor early American farmers, bourbon has survived Temperance, Prohibition and war to become one of the world's finest drinks. Unlike Scotch, it is made from 51% corn, aged in new, charred oak barrels and is made in America

RYE

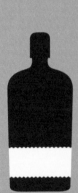

For whisky to be called rye in America it must be made from a mash of no less than 51% rye but in Canada no such laws were set and Canadian rye can be labelled as such even if the corn to rye ratio is as high as 9:1. Like bourbon, it is aged in new oak barrels and the same alcohol percentage rules apply

JAPANESE WHISKEY

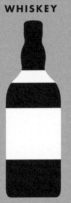

Japanese makers are now setting the whisky world alight, too: a Yamazaki Single Malt Sherry Cask 2013 was named the best in the world in the Whisky Bible 2015. Distilleries have been going for some 90 years, crafting a variety of malts and blends, and are now famed for their experimentation

TENNESSEE WHISKY

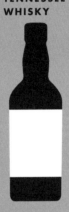

Straight bourbon made in the state of Tennessee but makers such as Jack Daniels claim they need to make the distinction, as theirs is the only whisky where the spirit goes through a charcoal filtering process

4. DISTILLATION

The mix is boiled and because alcohol vaporises at a lower temperature it is released quicker than the water, which is then condensed and collected as alcohol. The process is done several times to make a distillation of around 70%

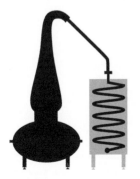

5. MATURATION

It's the storage in oak casks that give whisky its mellow flavour and distinctive colour (Scotch, for example, needs a minimum of three years). Old sherry or wine casks are traditionally used to 'finish' whiskies

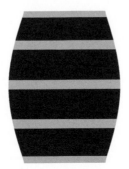

6. BLENDING & BOTTLING

Single malt is a barley whisky from one distillery although it will be blended from many different casks to give the final, desired flavour and colour. The alcohol level is then diluted to a strength of between 40% and 46% before bottling

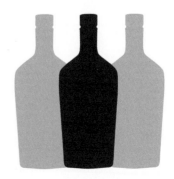

—

VODKA: AN ICY SHOT

For something that is best served straight out of the freezer, boy does vodka burn as it slips down the hatch. But, it wasn't always so.

Fermented from grain (usually wheat or rye, or vegetables such as potatoes), this potently pure alcohol originated in Eastern Europe, sometime around the 8th and 9th centuries. Both Poland and Russia claim it as their own, but regardless of its exact birthplace, it is certain that early versions of the drink were relatively weak, only reaching around 14% alcohol (similar to wine), compared to the 40% we see today, because the liquid was only fermented rather than distilled. Rudimentary distillation techniques in 16th-century Poland saw alcohol levels climb, industrial distilling began in the 18th century, and 100 years later new technology saw the appearance of vodka distilled to the clear liquid we know and love.

Russia's vodka production followed similar suit but legend has it here that the first recipe was concocted by a Moscow monk, who called the fiery shot 'bread wine' and 'burning wine'. Today vodka is produced around the world, but some of the best is found in Sweden, Finland, Estonia and Lithuania along the aptly titled 'Vodka Belt'.

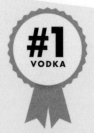

Vodka is the world's top-selling spirit

The word vodka comes from the Russian 'voda' and roughly translates as 'little water'

Vodka is best drunk ice-cold and thanks to its high alcohol content remains liquid when stored in the freezer

James Bond gave vodka a sophisticated boost with his signature drink of a Vodka Martini, shaken not stirred

IS VODKA BLAND?

A staple in many cocktails to up the proof without affecting the flavour (from Cosmos to Moscow Mules), vodka is often overlooked as a drink in its own right. But just as other clear, unaged drinks are having their day, such as malt spirit or 'white dog' (juvenille whiskies), seemingly 'neutral' vodkas are worth rescuing from the drinks cabinet. This naked spirit can taste of anything from citrus fruits and ripe apples to smoke and pepper, and is appreciated for its 'clean', smooth heat in the throat

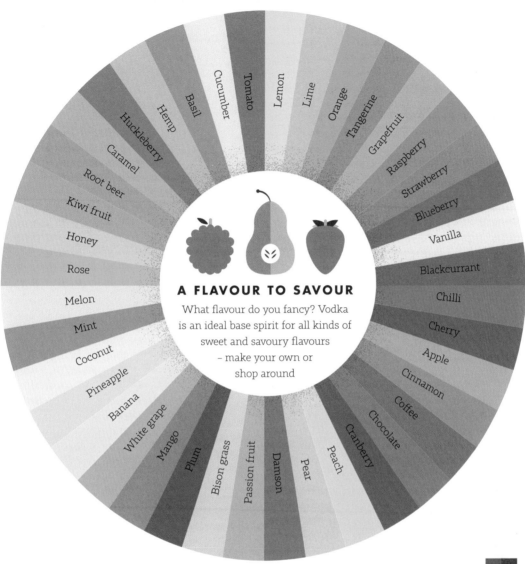

A FLAVOUR TO SAVOUR

What flavour do you fancy? Vodka is an ideal base spirit for all kinds of sweet and savoury flavours – make your own or shop around

Tomato · Cucumber · Basil · Hemp · Huckleberry · Caramel · Root beer · Kiwi fruit · Honey · Rose · Melon · Mint · Coconut · Pineapple · Banana · White grape · Mango · Plum · Bison grass · Passion fruit · Damson · Pear · Peach · Cranberry · Chocolate · Coffee · Cinnamon · Apple · Cherry · Chilli · Blackcurrant · Vanilla · Blueberry · Strawberry · Raspberry · Grapefruit · Tangerine · Orange · Lime · Lemon

IN CASE OF EMERGENCY

Traditionally vodka was used for medicinal purposes, it can be rubbed on feverish chests, and, like all alcohol, makes a good antiseptic

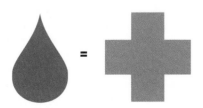

BOTTOMS UP!

While inoffensive vodka might have become the shooter of choice for those looking to get their alcohol fix quick, good vodka is best sipped and savoured. Never say 'nostrovia!' to a Russian, either, it doesn't mean cheers but is a thank you for a drink or meal, instead try 'za zdarovye' which means 'to health!'

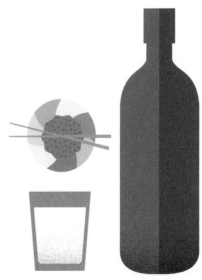

211

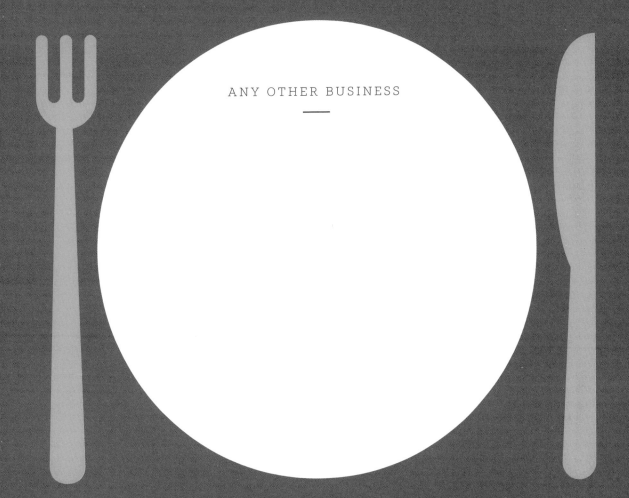

ANY OTHER BUSINESS

———

—

CONVERSION CHARTS: YOUR ESSENTIAL CHEAT SHEET

With so many ways to measure out our ingredients it's easy to get confused, but not anymore! Make sure you stick to the same measurement for a whole recipe and digital scales are a must for baking, which requires precise measurements for the perfect result. An oven thermometer is an equally good investment to make sure the inside of your cooker reflects the temperature on the dial.

OVEN TEMPERATURE

°C	°C (fan)	°F	GAS MARK
140°C	120°C	275°C	1
150°C	130°C	300°C	2
170°C	150°C	325°C	3
180°C	160°C	350°C	4
190°C	170°C	375°C	5
200°C	180°C	400°C	6
220°C	200°C	425°C	7
230°C	210°C	450°C	8
240°C	220°C	475°C	9

WEIGHTS

IMPERIAL	METRIC
½ oz	15g
1 oz	30g
2 oz	55g
3 oz	85g
4 oz	115g
5 oz	140g
6 oz	170g
7 oz	200g
8 oz	225g
9 oz	250g
10 oz	285g
11 oz	315g
12 oz	340g

You will need:
Digital scales
Oven thermometer
American cup
Measuring jug
Tape measure

214

1CUP

1/2

1/4

LIQUIDS

IMPERIAL	AMERICAN	METRIC
-	½ teaspoon	2.5ml
-	1 teaspoon	5ml
-	1 tablespoon	15ml
1 fl oz	-	30ml
2 fl oz	¼ cup	55ml
4 fl oz	½ cup	115ml
8 fl oz	1 cup	225ml
16 fl oz	1 American pint	470ml
20 fl oz	2½ cups	570ml
32 fl oz	1 quart (2 pints)	910ml
35 fl oz	-	1 litre

IMPERIAL	METRIC
1 inch	2.5cm
2 inches	5cm
3 inches	7.5cm
4 inches	10cm
5 inches	12.5cm
6 inches	15cm
7 inches	17.5cm
8 inches	20cm
9 inches	23cm
10 inches	25.5cm

LENGTHS

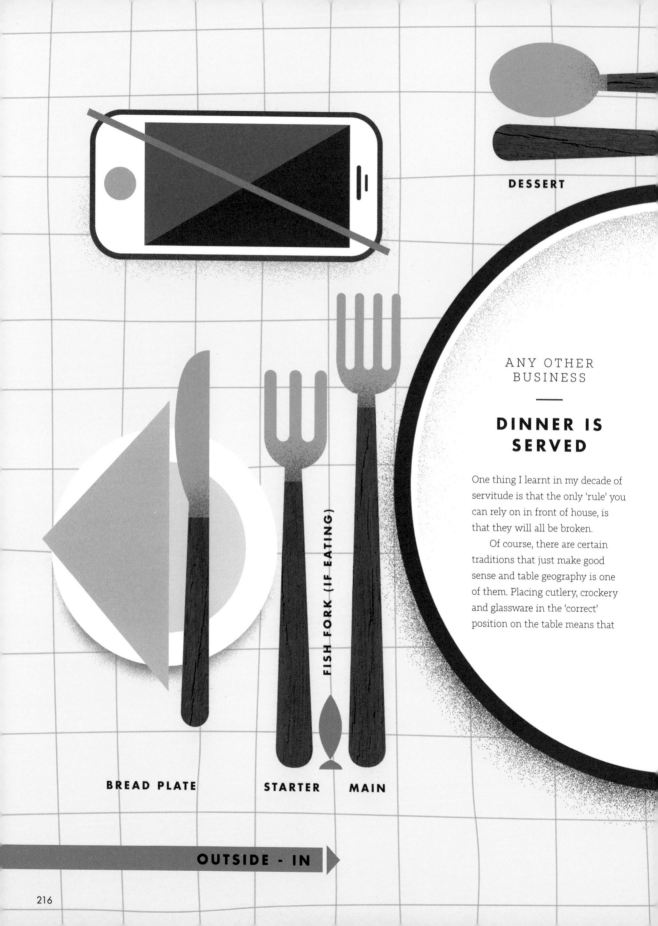

DESSERT

ANY OTHER
BUSINESS

—

DINNER IS
SERVED

One thing I learnt in my decade of
servitude is that the only 'rule' you
can rely on in front of house, is
that they will all be broken.

Of course, there are certain
traditions that just make good
sense and table geography is one
of them. Placing cutlery, crockery
and glassware in the 'correct'
position on the table means that

FISH FORK (IF EATING)

BREAD PLATE   **STARTER**   **MAIN**

OUTSIDE - IN

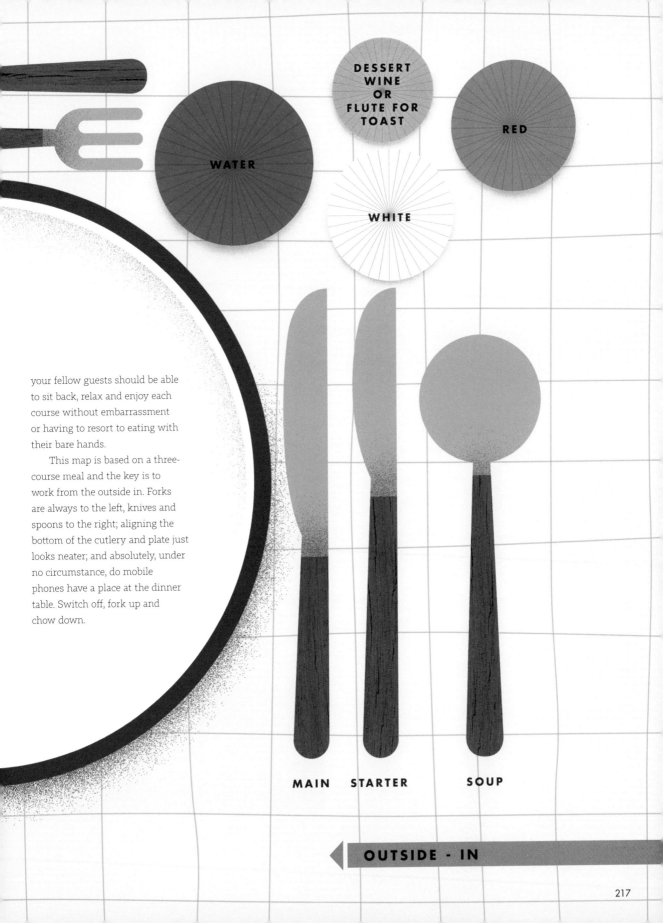

DESSERT
WINE
OR
FLUTE FOR
TOAST

WATER

RED

WHITE

your fellow guests should be able to sit back, relax and enjoy each course without embarrassment or having to resort to eating with their bare hands.

This map is based on a three-course meal and the key is to work from the outside in. Forks are always to the left, knives and spoons to the right; aligning the bottom of the cutlery and plate just looks neater; and absolutely, under no circumstance, do mobile phones have a place at the dinner table. Switch off, fork up and chow down.

MAIN   STARTER   SOUP

OUTSIDE - IN

EAT SEASONAL

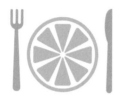

Not only do ingredients taste better fresher and less travelled, but they retain more of their valuable nutrients and are generally more pleasant to eat. Peaches are juicier, asparagus are sweeter, apples are crunchier.

Generally, you'll save a couple of coins too, if you eat the best of what's grown or reared locally. So make the most of what's available right now, reduce your food miles, and make shopping seasonally standard.

FRUIT	DEC	JAN	FEB	MAR	APR	MAY	JUN	JUL	AUG	SEP	OCT	NOV
APPLES	■	■	■	■	■	■	■	■	■	■	■	■
APRICOTS							■	■	■	■		
BLACKCURRANTS							■	■	■			
BLUEBERRIES							■	■				
BLACKBERRIES									■	■	■	■
BANANAS	■	■	■	■								
BLOOD ORANGES	■	■	■									
CLEMENTINES	■	■	■									■
CHERRIES							■	■	■	■		
CRANBERRIES	■											
DATES	■	■										
ELDERBERRIES										■	■	
FIGS									■	■		
GRAPES									■	■	■	
GOOSEBERRIES							■	■	■			
KIWI	■	■	■	■	■	■	■	■	■	■	■	■
LEMONS		■	■	■	■	■						
MELONS							■	■	■	■		
NECTARINES							■	■	■	■		
ORANGES	■	■	■									
PEARS	■	■	■									
PASSION FRUIT		■	■									
PEACHES							■	■	■	■		
PLUMS								■	■	■	■	■
PINEAPPLES		■	■									
PERSIMMONS	■											
POMEGRANATE	■	■	■	■	■							
QUINCES											■	
RHUBARB	■	■	■	■	■	■	■					
REDCURRANTS							■	■	■			
RASPBERRIES							■	■	■	■	■	
STRAWBERRIES						■	■	■	■	■		
SATSUMAS	■	■										
TANGERINE	■											■

VEGETABLES	DEC	JAN	FEB	MAR	APR	MAY	JUN	JUL	AUG	SEP	OCT	NOV
AUBERGINES							●	●	●	●	●	●
ASPARAGUS			●	●	●	●						
BEETROOT						●	●	●	●	●	●	●
BROAD BEANS								●	●			
BROCCOLI											●	●
BRUSSELS SPROUTS	●	●	●							●	●	●
CABBAGE	●	●	●	●	●	●	●	●	●	●	●	●
CARROTS	●	●	●	●	●	●	●	●	●	●	●	●
CAULIFLOWER	●	●	●									
CELERIAC										●	●	●
CELERY										●	●	●
CHICORY							●	●	●	●	●	●
CHILLIES								●	●	●	●	
COURGETTES							●	●	●	●	●	
FENNEL							●	●	●	●	●	●
FRENCH BEANS										●	●	●
GLOBE ARTICHOKES								●	●	●	●	
JERUSALEM ARTICHOKES	●	●	●	●								●
KALE	●	●	●	●								
KOHLRABI								●	●	●	●	
LEEKS	●	●	●	●	●							
LETTUCE LEAVES						●	●	●	●	●	●	
MOREL MUSHROOMS					●							
MARROW										●	●	
ONIONS				●								
PARSNIPS	●	●	●	●								●
POTATOES	●	●	●	●	●	●	●	●	●	●	●	●
PUMPKINS										●	●	
PEPPERS							●	●	●	●	●	●
PEAS					●	●	●	●	●	●	●	
RADISHES					●	●	●	●	●	●	●	
RUNNER BEANS							●	●	●	●	●	
SPINACH	●	●	●	●	●	●	●	●	●	●	●	●
SPRING ONIONS				●	●	●						
SWEDE	●	●	●									●
SAMPHIRE							●	●				
SUMMER SQUASH							●	●	●	●		
SWEETCORN								●	●	●		
SWISS CHARD							●	●	●	●	●	
TOMATOES							●	●	●	●	●	
TURNIP	●	●	●	●	●							
WILD MUSHROOMS	●	●										
WILD GARLIC				●	●	●						
WATERCRESS					●	●						

KNOW YOUR KNIVES

The recipe for the perfect meal extends far beyond your shopping basket of ingredients. From the pan you choose to cook in, to the plate you serve on, choosing the right tools for the job is just as essential. And, perhaps, no more so than when it comes to knives. You only really need four knives as far as I'm concerned – a chef's knife, paring knife, bread knife and filleting knife – but if you've got the space and budget then these 10 will really up your kitchen game. Always buy in person, rather than via the internet, as comfort when using the knife is just as important as the quality of the blade itself.

CHEF'S KNIFE

Don't be intimidated by its size. This large all-purpose knife (the most useful you will ever buy) makes quick work of chopping, crushing, dicing, slicing, mincing, scoring and julienne

FILLETING KNIFE

A long, thin and flexible blade designed to remove fillets of fish from the bone, as well as de-scale and de-skin

BONING KNIFE

Narrow (slightly shorter than a filleting knife) and with a certain amount of flexibility to help you get round all the nooks and crannies. Essential for creating clean cuts when boning and filleting pieces of meat

TOMATO KNIFE

Endlessly useful and forgiving – handy for everything from slicing tomatoes to segmenting an orange

PARING KNIFE

Just as every home should have a large knife, so should you have a small knife for more delicate jobs, from peeling to trimming

SHARPENING STEEL

A blunt knife is a dangerous one. Maintain control and keep your investments sharp with this specially designed rod, which can come as hard steel, diamond coated steel or ceramic. Place the tip of the steel, facing downwards, on a wooden chopping board and sharpen any knife in sweeping strokes away from you

BREAD KNIFE

A must for loaf lovers, this knife is serrated to ensure an even slice

CARVING KNIFE

Narrow and long enough to tackle roasted joints of meat and poultry

SANTOKU

Meaning 'three virtues' in Japanese, this broad, rigid and scalloped steel (lighter than a chef's knife) can slice, dice and mince; and is suitable for meat, fish and vegetables

CLEAVER

A large, thick blade ideal for cutting through bone but also rather useful for chopping big batches for herbs or mincing meat and fish

PEELING KNIFE

A short, curved, inflexible knife specially designed to peel vegetables and 'turning' them into barrel shapes

Just as people can be colour blind, a minority of people also experience taste blindness, and are unable to detect certain tastes, such as bitterness

Ever thought how delicious a sizzling steak or the clink of ice into a glass on a hot day sounds? Everything we hear is sending signals to our brain to complete our perception of taste

THE FIVE TASTES

Some people eat to fuel, ticking the protein, carbohydrate and five-a-day fruit and veg boxes, but those of us who eat for pleasure know that taste is a multisensory experience. It can provoke memories, it can cause us to pull faces and it can even inspire.

Part of our evolution and survival, taste is designed to help us to detect when something is potentially poisonous and unpleasant and helps us to crave the things our bodies naturally need, from sugary carbohydrates to salt and its essential minerals. It was ancient Greek philosopher Aristotle though who first distinguished between the basic tastes that we humans experience, starting with sweet and bitter, but it is now accepted that there are a further three: salty, sour and (the most recently discovered) umami.

For the past century or so it was thought that specific areas of the tongue detected each of these tastes – a 'tongue map' was created based on the research of a 20th-century German scientist, locating sweet at the tip, sour and salty along the sides and bitter at the back of the tongue – but that has since been proven wrong. Our taste buds can detect every type of taste, and it is our brain that finally identifies which one, along with the help of our other senses.

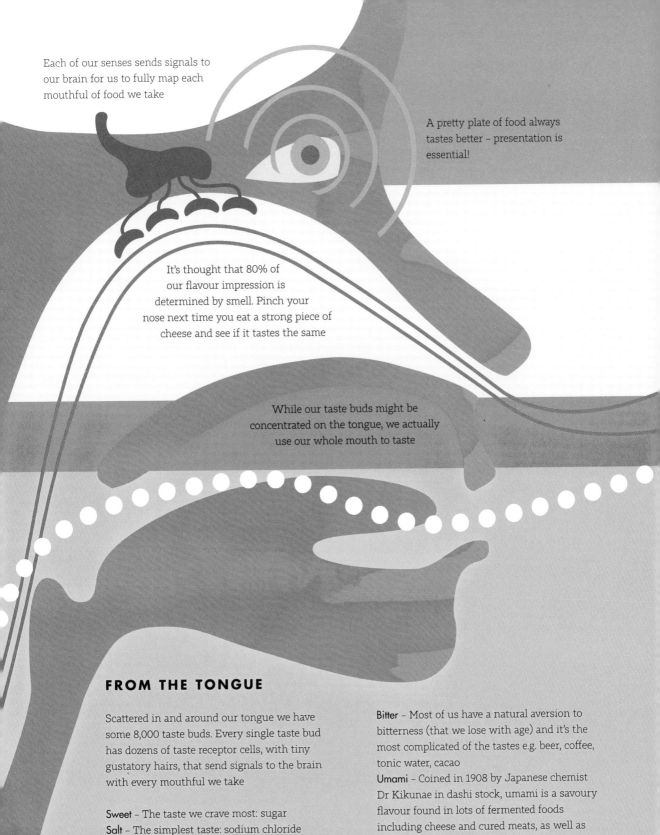

Each of our senses sends signals to our brain for us to fully map each mouthful of food we take

A pretty plate of food always tastes better – presentation is essential!

It's thought that 80% of our flavour impression is determined by smell. Pinch your nose next time you eat a strong piece of cheese and see if it tastes the same

While our taste buds might be concentrated on the tongue, we actually use our whole mouth to taste

FROM THE TONGUE

Scattered in and around our tongue we have some 8,000 taste buds. Every single taste bud has dozens of taste receptor cells, with tiny gustatory hairs, that send signals to the brain with every mouthful we take

Sweet – The taste we crave most: sugar
Salt – The simplest taste: sodium chloride
Sour – Acidic tastes such as citrus fruits

Bitter – Most of us have a natural aversion to bitterness (that we lose with age) and it's the most complicated of the tastes e.g. beer, coffee, tonic water, cacao
Umami – Coined in 1908 by Japanese chemist Dr Kikunae in dashi stock, umami is a savoury flavour found in lots of fermented foods including cheese and cured meats, as well as seaweed, mushrooms and tomatoes

FURTHER READING

Balinska, Maria. *The Bagel: The Surprising History of a Modest Bread* (New Haven and London: Yale University Press, 2008).

Bertinet, Richard. *Patisserie Maison* (London: Ebury Publishing, 2014).

Blythman, Joanna. *What to Eat* (London: Fourth Estate, 2012).

Bretherton, Caroline. *Step-by-Step Baking* (London: Dorling Kindersley, 2011).

Chandler, Jenny. *Pulse* (London: Pavilion Books, 2013).

Cloake, Felicity. *Perfect* (London: Fig Tree, 2011).

Cloake, Felicity. *Perfect Too* (London: Fig Tree, 2014).

Cross, Robert. *Classic 1000 Cocktail Recipes* (Berkshire: Foulsham, 2011).

Davidson, Alan. *The Oxford Companion to Food* (Oxford: Oxford University Press, 2014).

Edwards, Sarah Jane. *Chocolate Unwrapped* (London: Pavilion Books, 2010).

Gomi, Yuki. *Sushi at Home* (London: Penguin, 2013).

Grigson, Sophie. *The Soup Book* (London: Dorling Kindersley, 2009).

Harrar, Vanessa and Spence, Charles. 'The taste of cutlery: how the taste of food is affected by the weight, size, shape, and colour of the cutlery used to eat it', *Flavour* 2:21, (2013).

Holland, Mina. *The Edible Atlas* (Edinburgh: Canongate Books, 2014).

Joannides, Dino. *Semplice* (London: Preface Publishing, 2014).

Kimber, Edd. *The Boy Who Bakes* (London: Kyle Books, 2011).

Kinnaird, Dr Tim. *Perfecting Patisserie* (London: Apple Press, 2013).

Liger-Belair, Gerard. 'How Many Bubbles in Your Glass of Bubbly' *The Journal of Physical Chemistry* 118, (2014).

Manning, Anneka. *Mastering The Art of Baking* (Sydney: Murdoch Books, 2012).

Mathiot, Ginette. *I Know How to Cook* (London: Phaidon Press, 2009).

McCandless, David. *Information is Beautiful* (London: HarperCollins UK, 2012).

McCandless, David. *Knowledge is Beautiful* (London: HarperCollins UK, 2014).

McGee, Harold. *McGee on Food & Cooking: An Encyclopedia of Kitchen Science, History and Culture* (London: Hodder & Stoughton, 2004).

Melrose and Morgan. *Good Food for your Table: A Grocer's Guide* (London: Saltyard Books, 2014).

Presilla, Maricel E. *The Food of Latin America: Gran Cocina Latina* (New York: W.W. Norton & Company, 2012).

Roden, Claudia. *Book of Jewish Food* (London: Penguin, 1999).

Roden, Claudia. *Tamarind & Saffron* (London: Penguin, 2000).

Ramen, Ivan. *Love, Obsession and Recipes* (Bath: Absolute Press, 2014).

Segnit, Niki. *Flavour Thesaurus* (London: Bloomsbury Publishing, 2010).

Sitwell, William. *A History of Food in 100 Recipes* (London: HarperCollins UK, 2012).

Stein, Rick. *Fish & Shellfish* (London: Ebury Publishing, 2014).

Spaull, Susan and Burrell, Fiona. *Leiths Baking Bible* (London: Bloomsbury Publishing, 2012).

Spaull, Susan and Bruce-Gardyne, Lucinda. *Leiths Technique Bible* (London: Bloomsbury Publishing, 2012).

Stephenson, Tristan. *The Curious Bartender* (London: Ryland Peters & Small, 2013).

Wright, John. *The River Cottage Mushroom Handbook* (London: Bloomsbury Publishing, 2007).

WEBSITES

www.aboutoliveoil.org/consumption.html

www.aeb.org/farmers-and-marketers/industry-overview

www.agmrc.org/commodities__products/nuts/almond-profile/

www.agribenchmark.org/agri-benchmark/did-you-know/einzelansicht/artikel//tomatoes-are.html

www.atlanticsalmontrust.org

www.avocadocentral.com/about-hass-avocados/hass-mother-tree

www.bbcgoodfood.com

www.boell.de/sites/default/files/meat_atlas2014_kommentierbar.pdf

www.visual.ly/global-annual-ice-cream-consumption-top-five-countries-worldwide

www.britishcoffeeassociation.org/about_coffee/coffee_facts/

www.britishturkey.co.uk/facts-and-figures/christmas-stats-and-traditions.html

www.businessinsider.com/scoville-scale-for-spicy-food-2013-11?IR=T

www.cantontea.co.com

www.charmingitaly.com/different-types-of-pasta/

www.cipotato.org/potato/native-varieties/

www.cfaitc.org/factsheets/pdf/Avocados.pdf

www.chinahistoryforum.com/topic/2991-dim-sum-a-little-bit-of-heart-beginners-guide/

www.dairymoos.com/how-much-milk-do-cows-give/

www.deliaonline.com/home/conversion-tables.html

www.deliaonline.com/how-to-cook/preserves/ten-steps-to-jam-making.html

www.deliciousavocados.co.uk/nourishing

www.eattheseasons.co.uk

www.egginfo.co.uk/industry-data

www.fao.org

www.fao.org/agriculture/dairy-gateway/milk-and-milk-products/en/#.VUCYb7PF-PU

www.fao.org/ag/againfo/themes/images/meat/backgr_sources_data.jpg

www.fao.org/docrep/018/i3253e/i3253e.pdf

www.fishonline.org

www.foodpreservation.about.com/od/Preserves/a/High-And-Low-Pectin-Fruit.htm

www.foodtimeline.org/foodcandy.html#jellyjam

www.geniusofdrinking.com/drinking-101/vodka/trivia.html

www.huffingtonpost.co.uk/2011/12/06/our-christmas-dinner-takes-10-months-to-grow_n_1131850.html

www.ifr.ac.uk/science-society/spotlight/apples/

www.instantnoodles.org/report/index.html

www.jewishquarterly.org/issuearchive/articleadf.html?articleid=210

www.kitchenproject.com/history/sourdough.htm

kobikitchen.wordpress.com/2013/05/05/types-of-ramen/

www.livestrong.com/article/350652-percentage-of-water-in-fruits-vegetables/

www.lovepotatoes.co.uk

www.luckypeach.com/a-guide-to-the-regional-ramen-of-japan/

www.madehow.com/Volume-2/Tofu.html

www.msc.org/cook-eat-enjoy/fish-to-eat

www.nationalchickencouncil.org

www.nordicfoodlab.org

www.nourishedkitchen.com/how-to-make-a-sourdough-starter/

www.nutracheck.co.uk/media/docs/Christmas_day_the_naughty_way.pdf

www.nytimes.com/2003/12/31/dining/was-life-better-when-bagels-were-smaller.html

www.philadelphia.co.uk/Brand/History

www.saltassociation.co.uk/education/salt-health/salt-function-cells/

www.seriouseats.com/2013/09/the-serious-eats-guide-to-ramen-styles.html

www.soya.be/what-is-tofu.php

www.soyatech.com/soy_facts.htm

www.soyconnection.com/soy_foods/nutritional_composition.php

www.statista.com/statistics/279556/global-top-asparagus-producing-countries/

www.statista.com/statistics/268227/top-coffee-producers-worldwide/

www.telegraph.co.uk/men/the-filter/qi/8258009/QI-Quite-interesting-facts-about-the-cold.html

www.theguardian.com/science/blog/2013/oct/03/science-magic-jam-making

www.saffron.com/what.html

www.theguardian.com/science/blog/2010/aug/23/science-art-whisky-making

www.tea.co.uk

www.tea-info.co.uk

www.theatlantic.com/business/archive/2014/01/here-are-the-countries-that-drink-the-most-coffee-the-us-isnt-in-the-top-10/283100/

www.thewhiskyexchange.com

www.vegsoc.org

www.vodkafacts.net

www.vinepair.com

www.washingtonpost.com/blogs/wonkblog/wp/2014/08/06/the-rise-of-the-american-almond-craze-in-one-nutty-chart/

www.whisky.com

www.en.wikipedia.org/wiki/List_of_countries_by_apple_production

www.ricepedia.org/rice-as-a-crop/rice-productivity

www.en.wikipedia.org/wiki/Rice#cite_note-1

www.en.wikipedia.org/wiki/Tomato

www.winefolly.com

www.world-foodhistory.com/2011/07/history-of-pancakes.html

www.winemag.com

www.wineware.co.uk

www2.ca.uky.edu/enri/pubs/enri129.pdf

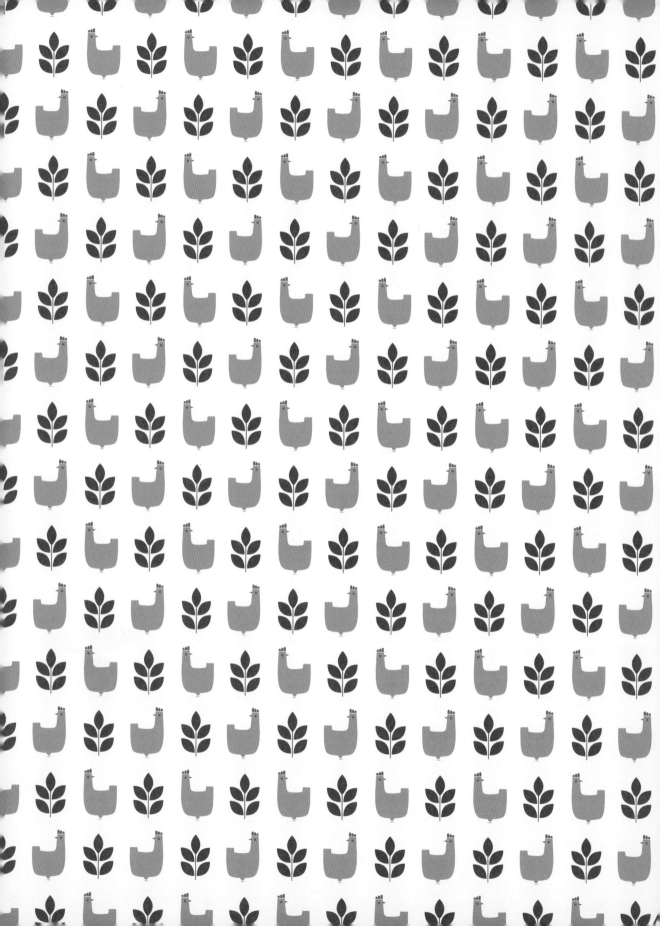